Advanced Genetic Counseling

Advanced Genetic Counseling
Theory and Practice

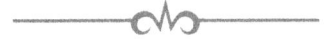

Barbara B. Biesecker, Kathryn F. Peters,
and Robert Resta

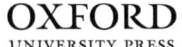

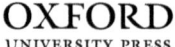

Oxford University Press is a department of the University of Oxford. It furthers the University's objective of excellence in research, scholarship, and education by publishing worldwide. Oxford is a registered trade mark of Oxford University Press in the UK and certain other countries.

Published in the United States of America by Oxford University Press
198 Madison Avenue, New York, NY 10016, United States of America.

© Oxford University Press 2019

All rights reserved. No part of this publication may be reproduced, stored in a retrieval system, or transmitted, in any form or by any means, without the prior permission in writing of Oxford University Press, or as expressly permitted by law, by license, or under terms agreed with the appropriate reproduction rights organization. Inquiries concerning reproduction outside the scope of the above should be sent to the Rights Department, Oxford University Press, at the address above.

You must not circulate this work in any other form
and you must impose this same condition on any acquirer.

Library of Congress Cataloging-in-Publication Data
Names: Biesecker, Barbara B., author. | Peters, Kathryn F., author. | Resta, Robert G., author.
Title: Advanced genetic counseling : theory and practice / Barbara B. Biesecker, Kathryn F. Peters, and Robert Resta.
Description: New York, NY : Oxford University Press, [2019] | Includes bibliographical references.
Identifiers: LCCN 2019017493 | ISBN 9780190626426 (pbk.) | ISBN 9780190626433(updf) | ISBN 9780190626440 (epub) | ISBN 9780190626457 (online)
Subjects: | MESH: Genetic Counseling | Professional-Patient Relations
Classification: LCC RB155.7 | NLM QZ 52 | DDC 362.196/ 042— dc23
LC record available at https://lccn.loc.gov/2019017493

CONTENTS

1. Introduction to Genetic Counseling   *1*
2. History of Genetic Counseling   *7*
3. Definitions and Goals of Genetic Counseling   *21*
4. Characteristics of Genetic Counseling Clients   *43*
5. Characteristics of Genetic Counselors   *69*
6. Applying Ethical Theories to Genetic Counseling Practice   *89*
7. Conflict of Interest and the Code of Ethics   *111*
8. Relational Genetic Counseling   *125*
9. Psychological Counseling Theories   *143*
10. Research in Genetic Counseling   *171*
11. Genetic Counseling in the Genomic Era   *187*

Appendix: Transcript of a Genetic Counseling Session   *201*
Index   *211*

CHAPTER 1

Introduction to Genetic Counseling

Any interaction between human beings is primarily a psychological interplay between the two parties. To paraphrase Charles Dickens from *A Christmas Carol*, this must be distinctly understood or nothing wonderful will come of the story we are going to relate. The words and behaviors of clients and counselors, as well as what they don't say or don't do, can simultaneously reveal and mask subtle clues to the psychological machinations of the human mind. A critical component of a genetic counselor's professional growth is to develop the counseling skills to be able to "read" patients to gain a better understanding of the psychological underpinnings of their hopes, dreams, fears, choices, actions, suffering, reactions, strengths, and apparent weaknesses, as well as their cognitive understanding of genetic information. Much of this ability comes with time and experience. But without basic counseling skills and insights, professional growth will be stunted.

The purpose of this book is to help you develop and expand some counseling skills that are key to your professional development. What you will not find in these pages are recurrence risks, comparisons of different prenatal screening strategies, the fine points of DNA sequencing or variant interpretation, or the details of metabolic biochemistry. While these are important technical components of genetic counseling, in and of themselves they are not the defining elements of genetic counseling.

We also want to emphasize that genetic counseling is not the same thing as genetic testing. Because much genetic counseling centers on genetic testing, there is a general tendency to conflate the two activities and sometimes to measure the effectiveness of genetic counseling based on test uptake. Instead we argue that the goals of genetic counseling are to help clients and their families adapt to the many effects of genetic disease or the risks of developing those diseases, improve their lives in sometimes small and sometimes large ways, and otherwise reinforce and strengthen their abilities to manage the medical and psychological and social impact of genetic disease on their lives and their families. Achieving these goals in any given case may or may not include the use of genetic testing, statistical information, or a detailed explanation of genetic variant interpretation.

Three basic assumptions underlie this text. The first assumption is that our patients and clients have the psychological wherewithal to adapt to whatever hereditary conditions they are confronting, though sometimes they may need to partner with genetic counselors and others to see and act on their strengths and abilities. The second assumption is that people are good and will strive to make the best decisions for themselves and their families. The third assumption is that each patient is unique and no one genetic counseling approach works for all situations, hence the need for genetic counselors to have multiple and flexible options in their genetic counseling toolkits.

Genetic counseling is as much about understanding yourself as it is about understanding your clients. Thus, this text addresses genetic counselors' self-awareness as much as it addresses ways of understanding and counseling our clients. Self-awareness of our implicit biases and the ways that our upbringing and social worlds have shaped our psyches and worldview is an extraordinarily difficult task that is an ongoing process for even the most skilled and seasoned genetic counselors.

Chapter 2 provides an historical overview of the practice and profession of genetic counseling. Why and how did the genetic counseling profession develop? How does it fit into the practice of medical genetics specifically and the delivery of medical services more broadly? What trends and socioeconomic factors have influenced the development of the profession and what factors will help shape its future? Why does the profession maintain the centrality of particular ethical values like autonomy and patient-centered care? How and why did genetic counseling expand beyond pediatric genetic disorders and reproduction? How does the past shape what genetic counselors do today? For genetic counselors to understand themselves professionally, they need to understand their history.

In Chapter 3 we assess the definition and goals of genetic counseling, which have changed and sharpened in their focus over time. We argue that education alone is inadequate to achieve the goals of genetic counseling. While education can be an important part of some genetic counseling sessions, what is more important is to understand how clients interpret that information through the prism of their personal experiences and sociocultural context and integrate that interpretation into coping with and adapting to genetic disease. If education alone were the goal of genetic counseling, clients would probably be better off reading a well-written pamphlet or a professionally designed app. Information recall by clients is at best a poor measure of the effectiveness of genetic counseling. Technical knowledge, in and of itself, does not help clients adapt to the myriad ramifications of genetic disease or improve their lives.

Chapter 4 looks at the characteristics of our clients and how they might impact the delivery and reception of genetic counseling services. Each client we meet is a unique individual, while at the same time clients may share traits that tie them to others—gender, age, ethnicity, health status, socioeconomic status, familial relationships (parent, child, extended family, etc.), and religion. Each of these can influence the shape, dynamics, and outcomes of a genetic counseling session. As important as it is to understand the way that client characteristics influence genetic counseling, it is equally important to understand how these same external factors influence the behaviors and beliefs of genetic counselors themselves.

Chapter 5 considers the psychological profile and makeup of genetic counselors. Genetic counselors chose the profession based on their interest in science and people, shaped by their life experiences that they bring to their learned craft. Exploring one's beliefs, assumptions, and biases can illuminate ways they emerge in interactions with patients. In the event that counselors' life experiences drew them to the profession, how are those assets to relationships with patients and when can they be a liability? This chapter addresses ways for genetic counselors to maximize their self-awareness and develop life-long learning practices to understand themselves as they present and respond to clients.

The genetic counseling profession and the field of bioethics by and large emerged at about the same time in the late 1960s and early 1970s. This may be more than just coincidence. Many of the issues and questions raised by bioethicists were faced daily by genetic counselors as new genetic technologies became integrated into medical care and continue to do so. Consequently, genetic counselors have been acutely aware of the ethical implications of genetic medicine and genetic technology. Chapter 6 discusses different ethical theories in the context of genetic counseling practice. Chapter 7 applies the theories within a discussion of professional ethical dilemmas that may arise within the context of conflicts of interest that genetic counselors face when they interact with patients, researchers, clinics, and privately owned laboratories.

Chapter 8 addresses one of the most intimidating and exciting aspects of genetic counseling—that is, counseling itself. A lack of confidence in one's counseling skills may be why genetic counselors tend to fill the counseling space with an overabundance of technical discussion. It is much easier to recite arcane information than it is to assess and implement effective ways to engage a client in a psychologically meaningful interaction. This chapter explores the development of that meaningful relationship. We examine the concept of relational genetic counseling and discuss different techniques for establishing a psychotherapeutic relationship with clients during the course of a single genetic counseling session.

Chapter 9 examines psychological counseling theories and how they apply to genetic counseling practice. Our clients face differing circumstances that cannot be informed by a single theory. Mastering counseling theories can lead to goal-directed psychotherapeutic genetic counseling that meets clients' needs, such as making a difficult decision or adapting to a health risk. Approaches to crisis and grief counseling are applied and differ from theoretically informed practices. The chapter provides concrete ways in which theories, such as cognitive-behavioral and person-centered approaches, can be used to enhance a client's ability to navigate a challenging circumstance and emerge stronger from the experience.

Research on genetic counseling, particularly evaluating its effectiveness, is critical to informing ways the genetic counseling profession needs to grow, stay relevant, and be useful to patients and to the larger system of medical care delivery. All of our psychotherapeutic and educational endeavors are for naught if they are not effective in helping clients. In Chapter 10 we discuss the science and theories behind decision-making and health behavior, and how they are critical to conducting research and applying the results of that research to improving the delivery of genetic counseling services. Counselors are encouraged to actively participate in research at any level that interests them. We share interesting questions that affect our clients and encourage counselors to generate data to inform effective novel practice delivery modes.

Genetic technology and testing are expanding at rates not dissimilar from Moore's Law. This provides a very bright—albeit challenging—future for genetic counselors and genetic counseling. In Chapter 11, we look at the ways that genomic medicine has impacted the practice and profession of genetic counseling. We consider how the practice and profession may need to change and adapt as genomic sequencing becomes a part of routine medical care.

We close the book with an appendix that contains a transcript of a theoretical genetic counseling session. We do not provide our own commentary on this transcript. Instead, we trust the readers of this book and their instructors to critically read the transcript in light of what you learned from reading this book. The counseling provided by the counselor has strengths and weaknesses, and we leave it to you to decide which is which, as well as to consider alternative ways that the counselor could have conducted the session. This provides a learning tool for a group or individual discussion of a counseling session from start to finish and to evaluate it on a line-by-line, detailed basis. We want this discussion to provide you with insights into how you might practice genetic counseling when you are alone in a room with a client or family and don't have an instructor or handbook available to tell you what to do next or how to do it.

We don't want students to emerge from their training programs as professional clones of each other or of their program directors, with everyone delivering genetic counseling in the same way. Instead, we beseech you to develop your own unique but adaptable genetic counseling style, and to have the skills, confidence, and strength to critically evaluate yourself and to continue to change your practice accordingly. We want you to be the best genetic counselor you can possibly be, not only for appreciating your self-worth but also so that clients and patients will receive the best care possible to improve their own lives and the lives of those around them. To do so, accept that learning professional counseling skills is a long-term investment and commit to engaging in life-long learning. Join a peer supervision group. If one does not exist where you practice, start one. We hope this book provokes your high-level thinking and sparks your ambition to achieve these outcomes. The future and hopes of the profession and practice of genetic counseling depend on you.

CHAPTER 2

History of Genetic Counseling

The history of genetic counseling as a clinical activity should be distinguished from the history of genetic counseling as a profession. These are two distinct but intertwined stories. The narrative described here primarily reflects how genetic counseling evolved in the United States. The US model of the clinical practice and of the profession has to varying degrees influenced the development of genetic counseling in other countries. Nonetheless, in each geographic region genetic counseling has more or less followed a unique path shaped by local medical, historical, sociocultural, and economic factors.

MEDICAL GENETICS, GENETIC COUNSELING, AND EUGENICS: A COMPLICATED SET OF RELATIONSHIPS

Genetic counseling as a clinical activity predates the genetic counseling profession by many decades. Genetic counseling, and ultimately the field of medical genetics, has its roots in human genetics, animal genetics, teratology, laboratory science, psychiatry, embryology, and obstetrics. Susan Lindee (2016) has convincingly demonstrated that studies of the atomic bomb survivors in Nagasaki and Hiroshima helped shape the field of medical genetics in the latter half of the twentieth century. However, there is little evidence that work on the health effects of the atomic bomb directly influenced the development of the genetic counseling profession.

Technical and clinical advances in genetic medicine were critical to the growth of medical genetics; the application of genetic technologies and medical genetic knowledge to patient care was critical to the practice of genetic counseling. To the extent that medical care is embedded into the larger socioeconomic milieu, so too has genetic counseling reflected the unique cultural, sociological, and historical web within which it is practiced. While many factors influenced the historical development of genetic counseling, eugenics served as its most direct and immediate ancestor.

The term "eugenics" was coined in the latter part of the nineteenth century by Francis Galton, a half-first cousin of Charles Darwin. Eugenics was primarily focused on using genetic information to solve perceived social problems such as poverty, mental illness, racial degeneration, and declining intelligence.

Eugenic philosophies and programs arose in the United States, Canada, and many European countries. The manifestations of eugenics varied with local socioeconomic factors, historical traditions, medical practices, and governmental policies. Broadly speaking, the eugenics movements in England and the United States had the greatest influences on the development and practice of genetic counseling and medical genetics. For further details on the development of eugenics and medical genetics in the United States and other countries, interested readers are referred to several excellent works by Diane Paul, Daniel Kevles, Alexandra Minna Stern, Nathaniel Comfort, and Peter Harper included in the reference list for this chapter, as well as the Genetics and Medicine Historical Network (https://genmedhist.eshg.org).

In 1909 Karl Pearson, a founding figure of modern statistical analysis and Galton's most famous and influential disciple, served as the editor of what was to be the first of several volumes of a publication called *The Treasury of Human Inheritance*, published under the auspices of the Frances Galton Laboratory for National Eugenics in London, England. The book was a compendium of photographs, radiological images, pedigrees, and clinical descriptions of a range of physical disorders such as cleft lip and palate, limb anomalies, hemophilia, and short stature, along with a few chapters on the genetics of behavioral phenotypes such as "ability" and "insanity" thrown in for good eugenic measure. *The Treasury* was the intellectual forebear of later seminal clinical genetics textbooks such as David Smith's *Recognizable Patterns of Human Malformation* (1970), Josef Warkany's *Mental Retardation and Congenital Malformations of the Central Nervous System* (1975), and Robert Gorlin's and Jens Pindborg's *Syndromes of the Head and Neck* (1964).

Pearson felt that *The Treasury* would be of equal interest to "the pathologist, biologist, or eugenist" though the primary goal of the work "was the scientific maintenance of the health, physical and mental, of the nation." The clinical information in the book was intended to enable "more emphatic advice to be given" in what, from a twenty-first-century perspective, appears to be a mix of eugenic goals on a population scale and genetic counseling on a familial scale.

Two textbooks helped lay the groundwork for the development of the field of medical genetics and the practice of genetic counseling (although the term "genetic counseling" had not yet been coined when these books were published): Lawrence Snyder's *Principles of Heredity* (1935) and J. A. Fraser Robert's *An Introduction to Medical Genetics* (1940). These texts focused primarily on clinical and theoretical aspects of genetics and as such represent the earliest signs of at least a partial separation of medical genetics from classical eugenics.

By the 1930s, many scientists and physicians became disenchanted with classical eugenics, a shift reinforced by the horrors of Nazi Germany. However, as Diane Paul has shown (Paul, 1995; Paul, 1998), although many geneticists distanced themselves from certain eugenic practices and philosophies, they still readily supported some eugenic goals. Indeed, the first medical genetics clinic in the United States was founded in the 1940s in Winston-Salem, North Carolina, by C. Nash Herndon and William Allan. As Nathaniel Comfort (2012) has shown, eugenics was very much on the mind of these two geneticists when they established their department at the Bowman Gray School of Medicine. The Dight Institute of Human Genetics at the University of Minnesota, where Sheldon Reed practiced, was established with funds from Charles Dight, a multimillionaire with a strong interest in eugenics. Lee Dice, the founder of the Heredity Clinic at the University of Michigan, wrote promotional articles for the clinic with titles like "U. of M. Heredity Clinic Seeks to Improve Human Breed."

This is not to imply the simplistic model that medical genetics was simply eugenics ethically spiffed up and medicalized. Rather, it is naive to assume that the genetics world made a clean break from eugenics immediately after World War II. Eugenic philosophies lingered for decades after the 1940s. The development and practice of medical genetics was directly influenced by eugenics because of the overlap of interest in congenital anomalies and developmental disabilities as well as a reaction to the shocking eugenic practices of Nazi Germany (which, to some extent, were initially based on American and British eugenics). Understanding the eugenic roots of medical genetics—and hence genetic counseling—also helps put in historical perspective the eugenic criticisms of medical genetics that have been leveled against it since the introduction of prenatal diagnosis in the 1970s and 1980s.

The occurrence of two epidemics of birth defects—congenital rubella syndrome and thalidomide embryopathy—were critical to the developing field of dysmorphology. Somewhat ironically, both of these syndromes are decidedly nongenetic, caused as they are by environmental factors—the rubella virus and the pharmaceutical thalidomide (which, having failed when marketed as Grippex as a treatment for upper respiratory infections, was rebranded as Contergan and marketed as a treatment for pregnancy-related nausea, and went on to become one of the most successful—and tragic—prescription drugs ever). Many early medical geneticists had little formal training in genetics; instead, embryology and pediatrics were their primary skill sets (Löwy 2017), which served them well in proving that thalidomide and rubella were teratogenic agents. The study of embryopathy was also critical to understanding the pathology of the many genetic disorders in which normal embryonic development of fetal anatomy is altered or disrupted.

Victor McKusick at Johns Hopkins in Baltimore published the first comprehensive catalog of Mendelian diseases in *Mendelian Inheritance in Man* in 1966, without illustrations or photographs. McKusick is often called the "father of medical genetics" because, starting in the 1960s and continuing for about four decades, his program trained many national and international medical geneticists. McKusick's catalog went through many editions before it eventually became available online (https://www.omim.org); it is known as *OMIM* to today's genetic counselors and medial geneticists.

JOURNALS

Some of the primary outlets for publication of medical genetics articles were eugenic-based journals. The journal *Annals of Eugenics* was founded by Karl Pearson in 1924 and was one of the few publications that devoted space to articles about medical genetics (in 1954, the journal changed its name to *Annals of Human Genetics*). Throughout the 1950s, *Eugenics Quarterly*, the official journal of the American Eugenics Society, served as an important outlet for the publication of medical genetics research. Indeed, in this period, *Eugenics Quarterly* nearly quadrupled its number of subscribers from 281 to 1,033 (for comparison in its professional role, this is roughly the same number of subscribers to the *Journal of Genetic Counseling* at its debut in 1992). By 1968, the journal changed its name to *Social Biology*.

The *American Journal of Human Genetics* was also an important source of articles about medical genetics. First appearing in 1949, it was, and still is, the official journal of the American Society of Human Genetics (ASHG, founded in 1948). Although never a significant source of eugenic articles, many of the ASHG's founding members were also members of the American Eugenics Society—Wickliffe Draper, Samuel J. Holmes, Frederick Osborn, Carleton Coon, Ernest Hooton, Madge Macklin, William Allan (an annual

William Allan Award is still awarded annually to an ASHG member for significant contributions to the study of human genetics), C. Nash Herndon, William Allan, Sheldon Reed (who coined the term "genetic counseling"), Lee Dice, and Laurence Snyder (the author of the first genetics text that addressed medical issues).

The first publication devoted specifically to medical genetics was the *Journal of Medical Genetics*, published in the United Kingdom, which first appeared in September 1964. The topics covered in the articles in the first few volumes would not be out of place in a genetics journal published today. There is barely a whiff of eugenics in its content. As was typical for this and other medical genetics journals to come later (*Clinical Genetics, American Journal of Medical Genetics*), articles focused on the clinical and laboratory aspects of medical genetics; articles specifically about genetic counseling were few and far between.

THE PRACTICE OF GENETIC COUNSELING

Even to this day, very little research has been conducted on what actually transpires during a genetic counseling session, whether it is conducted by a physician, genetic counselor, or other health care professional. Thus, it is difficult to compare and contrast the content of genetic counseling sessions when conducted by individuals with differing training.

The earliest medical genetics and genetic counseling texts by Sheldon Reed (1955) and J. A. Fraser Roberts (1940) acknowledged the importance of emotional and psychological factors in the conduct of genetic counseling. But as much as textbooks and journal articles can be a measure of the practice of genetic counseling, a reasonable generalization can be made that genetic counseling conducted by medical geneticists focused primarily on establishing diagnoses and determining recurrence risks and strategies for dealing with both—ensuring proper medical guidance for individuals affected by genetic diseases as well as means of reducing the risk of, or avoiding the birth of, another affected child. In contrast, genetic counseling, when conducted by masters-level professional genetic counselors, shares a focus on information sharing, but also strives to include a counseling component that specifically addresses the emotional and psychological issues raised by being affected by or at risk for genetic diseases as well as walking with the client through the process of decision making when appropriate.

More serious integration of the psychological component of genetic counseling began in the late 1970s with the work of Seymour Kessler, the former director of the genetic counseling training program at the University of California, Berkeley. Kessler was by no means the first author to write seriously about the psychological and psychotherapeutic aspects of genetic counseling. In the early 1960s, Robert Tips and co-authors published several seminal papers that acknowledged and explored the psychological and social component of genetic counseling. The social work implications of genetic counseling were also recognized in the 1960s in publications by Sylvia Schild, and eventually a book in 1984 by Schild and Rita Beck Black, *Social Work and Genetics: A Guide for Practice*. The year 1984 also saw the publication of Alan Emery's *Psychological Aspects of Genetic Counselling*.

An influential article that helped introduce psychotherapy into the practice of genetic counseling was written by the psychiatrist Steven Targum in 1981. Deborah Eunpu in 1997 wrote the first article by a genetic counselor that systematically examined the role of psychotherapy in genetic counseling.

But it was Kessler, both in publication and in running the genetic counseling training program at Berkeley, who was most critical to the integration of counseling skills into genetic counseling practice and research. Beginning in 1981, Dr. Kessler produced a dozen or so seminal papers under the broad general title of "Psychological Aspects of Genetic Counseling" (Resta, 2000). These papers focused on the counseling content of a genetic counseling session and emphasized the importance of basic counseling skills in working with genetic counseling patients.

These publications laid the groundwork for the 2000 publication of *Psychosocial Genetic Counseling* by Jon Weil, Kessler's successor as head of the genetic counseling training program at Berkeley. This was the first comprehensive text aimed at integrating counseling skills into all aspects of genetic counseling. Other genetic counseling texts have since been published that have built on the work of Kessler and Weil (e.g., Evans and Harper, 2006).

THE GENETIC COUNSELING PROFESSION AND ITS RELATIONSHIP WITH MEDICAL GENETICS

The history of genetic counseling in America is well told by Alex Stern, and much of what follows draws from her work (Stern 2012). The genetic counseling profession has its roots in many social trends, including the feminist movement, expanding career opportunities for women, the availability of safe and legal abortion, the gradual disappearance of a paternalistic patient care philosophy, the growth of patient-centered medical care, recognition of the importance of understanding the patient as a person rather than as a disease entity, and delayed childbearing, along with advances in medical technology such as karyotyping, cell culturing techniques, ultrasonography, electrophoresis, and amniocentesis.

The first genetic counseling training program was established at Sarah Lawrence College, a liberal arts school just north of New York City. The program's founder (Melissa Richter) and the first director (Joan Marks) were, respectively, a psychologist and a medical social worker by training. Neither had formal training in medical genetics; at the time there were no medical geneticists on the regular Sarah Lawrence faculty, nor was there a medical center affiliated with the college. In order for students to be properly trained in medical genetics, the training program established relationships with medical genetics departments in the greater New York area. It was not uncommon for graduating students to be hired at the medical centers where they had interned.

Initially, at least, many genetic counselors (overwhelmingly female) worked under the direct supervision of (usually male) medical geneticists. Although many genetic counselors were highly skilled, initially many were treated as glorified clerical staff who organized clinics, obtained medical records, and assisted physicians during exams, but had fewer opportunities for independent practice. Over time, genetic counselors and medical geneticists became mutually dependent on one another to ensure the smooth flow of patient care and busy clinics. However, many of these bright, highly educated counselors sought positions with greater independence that allowed better utilization of their skills that did not necessarily involve a medical geneticist sitting in the room with them. It did not take long for many graduates to create new positions for themselves that required an appreciation for the psychological and social issues of genetic disorders. Thus, masters-trained genetic counselors established themselves as professionals who addressed the social needs, emotional issues, and educational concerns, along with some of the medical matters, of their clients.

As new opportunities opened up in the field of genetics that were not necessarily within the purview of traditional medical genetics, genetic counselors were quick to seize the employment opportunity. This is best exemplified by the introduction of prenatal diagnosis via amniocentesis in the 1970s, followed in the 1980s by maternal serum screening for neural tube defects and aneuploidy, ultrasonography, and chorionic villus sampling. The evolving standard of care was that all women who were considering prenatal testing should undergo genetic counseling. This opened up enormous employment potential as the numbers of amniocenteses increased dramatically. The training and relatively low salaries of genetic counselors made them the ideal professionals to provide genetic counseling to the tens of thousands of women who were considering prenatal diagnosis. And, over time, many genetic counselors found themselves interacting primarily with obstetricians and radiologists rather than medical geneticists. Similar trends followed as genetic counselors expanded their services to include neurology, psychotherapy, epidemiology, and, in the last few decades, oncology, cardiology, and laboratory practice (see Figure 2.1). While the relationship between genetic counselors and medical geneticists always remained important, for many genetic counselors it became increasingly common to only rarely interact with medical geneticists in their practices.

Genetic counselors and medical geneticists shared an accreditation organization—the American Board of Medical Genetics (ABMG)—and took some of the same written examinations when professional accreditation was instituted in 1982. Beginning in 1991 the two professional groups started to separate from one another (Resta 2010). This was driven in part by practical issues. The ABMG wished to become part of the American College of Medical Specialties (ACMS). However, ACMS would not admit nonphysicians. Thus, in order to join the ACMS, the ABMG had to eliminate all master's-level genetic counselors from its constituency. This required a vote of the membership, a controlling minority of which were genetic counselors. An at times bitter debate among the ABMG membership arose, but eventually the issue was voted on and the result was in favor of removing genetic counselors from the ABMG.

This led to the establishment of the American Board of Genetic Counseling (ABGC) in 1993, which then became the sole certifying

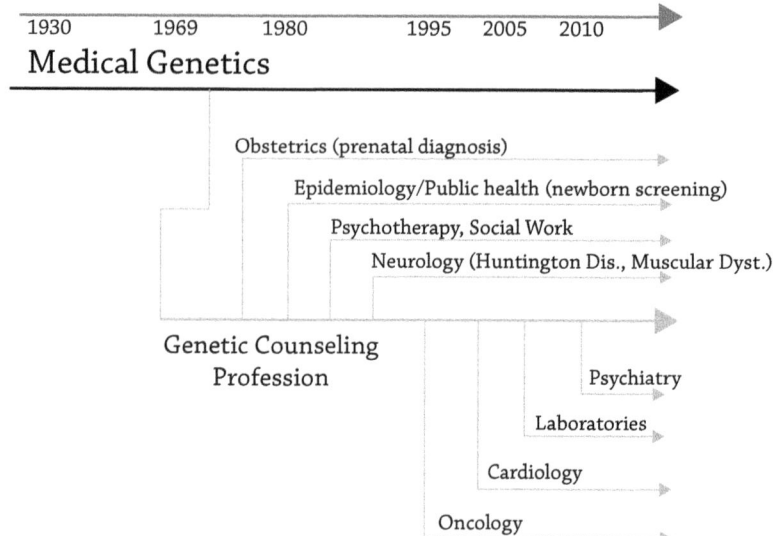

Figure 2.1 Timeline for The Professional Expansion of Genetic Counselors

program for masters-level genetic counselor in the United States. For the first time, genetic counselors were no longer dependent on medical geneticists for professional certification. This was a critical step for the genetic counseling profession to assert its independence and its value to the overall delivery of medical services.

Not to make too fine a point of distinction, but the birth of the genetic counseling profession had almost no direct connection to eugenics, whereas medical genetics was more intimately connected to eugenicists and eugenic philosophy. This is not to imply the simplistic argument that medical geneticists subscribe to a eugenic philosophy but genetic counselors do not. Genetic counselors still routinely use pedigrees—the primary tool and symbol of eugenics—in their daily practice. And genetic counselors are not immune to the eugenic criticisms that have been raised about the practice of genetic counseling by people with disabilities, their families, and their supporters.

The First Genetic Counseling Training Programs

The initial Sarah Lawrence College student cohort comprised older students looking for career training in midlife, and the program's interdisciplinary curriculum focused on the science of human genetics (Marks and Richter 1976). "Supervised clinical traineeships" organized at area hospitals served as practicums into the social and psychological aspects of genetic disorders. As the program matured, the need was established for more formal training in counseling skills necessary to address the psychological and social concerns of genetics clinic patients. In 1976, a course was added to the Sarah Lawrence program on counseling based on the philosophy of Carl Rogers (Marks 1993).

During the 1970s other universities began master's-level genetic counseling training programs. One particularly notable program, the training program at Berkeley, emerged independently from the Sarah Lawrence program in 1973. The Berkeley program was founded on problem-based learning and clinical experience. In addition to coursework in genetics, the program also sought to expose students in a concrete way to the psychological and social aspects of living with and making decisions about genetic conditions, and then teach students the psychological and social counseling skills they need to support people facing issues related to genetic conditions. This involved several educational innovations that continue to the present. First, as preparation for genetic counseling clinical rotations in the second year, each first-year student completes a field placement with a health or social service agency serving individuals with disabilities or facing long-term health care issues. This provides experience working as part of a health care team with individuals and families and develops awareness of community resources. Second, clinical supervision, analogous to the supervision given to students training in clinical psychology/psychiatry, was instituted. In addition, the program required that students tape-record counseling sessions for review and analysis with supervisors (Kessler, 2000). In the early 1990s, study of the impact of ethnocultural issues on the genetic counseling process was included as a major training element. Initially, the Berkeley program was faulted as being "too psychological and social." However, time has shown that the emphasis on the psychological and social aspects of genetic diagnoses is pivotal to genetic counseling training and practice.

In 1974, various faculty members from the founding genetic counseling training programs met with students and graduates to begin the discussion of formalized training goals and expectations for the genetic counseling profession (Walker 1998). Additional meetings centered on master's-level genetic counselor training and practice were held in 1976, 1979, and 1989 and resulted in the establishment of formal recommendations for training and practice in genetic counseling (Walker et al. 1990). Together, these meetings are known as the "Asilomar meetings" because three of the four meetings occurred at California's conference grounds in Asilomar. In 1992, the genetic counseling curriculum guidelines were again revisited and recommendations were made to enhance graduate education in human variation and diversity, genetic discrimination, nondirectiveness, and genetic screening policy (Biesecker et al. 1993). In 1996, the ABGC established formal genetic counseling practice and graduate training requirements based on twenty-seven practice-based competencies (Fiddler et al. 1996; Fine et al. 1996).

As of June 2018, there are forty-three genetic counseling training programs accredited by the Accreditation Counsel for Genetic Counseling (ACGC) in North America, and another six in development. There are also some twenty-five to thirty or so programs in Europe, Asia, Australia, the Philippines, South Africa, and Cuba. The ABGC has certified more than four thousand genetic counselors.

Professional Growth

The establishment of a professional society was a powerful means for masters-trained genetic counselors to achieve prestige and compensation at a professional level (Kenen 1984). Although a number of genetic counselors had joined the American Society of Human Genetics, as early as 1973, masters-level genetic counselors were discussing the notion of forming a unique professional society (Heimler 1997). It was not until the late 1970s, however, that the idea took shape. In 1977, a group of students from Sarah Lawrence College, along with a number of working genetic counselors, hosted a series of gatherings to discuss the issue, and by fall 1978, a core of masters-trained genetic counselors had begun to organize.

Three issues regarding the proposed national society were debated (Heimler 1997). First, there was the issue of the name. Some professionals preferred the title "genetic associate" whereas others lobbied for "genetic counselor." Interestingly, there was considerable resistance from the medical genetics community against the use of the title "genetic counselor" for nonphysicians. As Charles Epstein, a prominent medical geneticist, explained:

> Whether they be basic geneticists (Ph.D.), public health nurses, social workers, or genetic associates, they are certainly capable of providing valuable assistance and of carrying out many of the functions that are part of the overall counseling situation. Nevertheless, their ultimate value in counseling and ability to function depends on the presence of the responsibility-taking medical geneticist-physician-counselor, and for this reason I do not regard these individuals as "genetic counselors." Although this might appear to be merely a semantic distinction, there are reasons to argue otherwise. Titles have their own connotations, both to persons who hear them and to those who bear them. To us, the term "genetic counselor" connotes one who is capable of giving genetic counseling, with all that it entails. It is my contention, and I am prepared to be proven wrong, that except in the rarest of instances, non-medically trained individuals are not so prepared. Further, in view of the recent trend toward the establishment of training programs for allied health personnel . . . it must be explicitly stated that such programs in the area of genetics are not training genetic counselors—associates, assistants, aides, collaborators, yes; counselors, no! (Epstein 1973, pp. 43–44)

However, after working with genetic counselors for several years, Dr. Epstein developed a deep respect for their skills and contributions and became among their strongest supporters.

The founders of the society, however, did not agree with these sentiments. Rather, they viewed their masters-level training and practice as complementary to, yet distinct from, the practice of medical genetics. The term "associate" connoted a dependence on medical geneticists that the society's founding members did not countenance. In short, they believed that "any other title (than genetic counselor) would diminish the definition of the profession" (Heimler 1997, p. 320). Hence, the committee chose "genetic counselor" for the title of their profession.

The second point of contention was the membership criteria (Heimler 1997). The issue was whether or not non-master's-trained individuals providing genetic counseling should have full, voting membership in the society. This debate, as well as the debate over the name, represents beginning efforts of genetic counselors to distinguish themselves from their physician colleagues. After considerable debate, the committee decided on a tiered system of membership, with full membership reserved "for persons with a Master's or PhD degree in human genetics from a recognized genetic counseling program or in a related field" (Heimler 1997, p. 332).

The third point of contention was how national representation would be guaranteed in the society. At the time of the society's conception, there were fewer than 250 masters-trained genetic counselors in the United States, working in a variety of geographic areas. The committee decided to have regional representatives from each of six geographic regions.

In June 1979, Lorraine Suslak, Niecee Singer, Sylvia Rubin, Hody Tannenbaum, Luba Djurdjinovic, Evelyn Lilienthal, Phyllis Klass, Deborah Eunpu, and Audrey Heimler finished drafting the fledgling society's bylaws, and the National Society of Genetic Counselors (NSGC) became a reality. Since that time, the NSGC has grown to over four thousand members. It has sponsored nearly forty national educational conferences and provided financial support for research in genetic counseling. The NSGC has also sought to influence local and national policies affecting its members by sending representatives to federal and local hearings, as well as developing formal policy statements regarding genetic counseling issues.

NSGC now sees its mission as advancing "the various roles of genetic counselors in health care by fostering education, research, and public policy to ensure the availability of quality genetic services." This mission statement would likely meet with the approval of its founders. After four decades the group continues to play a critical role for the genetic counseling profession, but it will thrive in the future only if the next generation of genetic counselors (i.e., you!) become actively involved in volunteering to fill the many roles, large and small, needed to run a professional organization.

The *Journal of Genetic Counseling*, the official NSGC publication, was founded in 1992 with Deborah Eunpu, a founding member of the NSGC, as editor-in-chief. This was the first genetics journal devoted primarily to psychological, social, emotional, familial, and professional aspects of genetic counseling. This journal is run primarily for and by the genetic counseling profession. (The similarly named journal *Genetic Counseling* began publishing under this name in 1990—prior to that it was called *Journal de Génétique Humaine*—but it focuses primarily on medical rather than counseling issues.)

In 2005, the NSGC established a committee to formulate a new definition of genetic counseling that reflected the modern practice of genetic counseling that was derived from but also distinct from the definition crafted thirty-five years earlier by an ASHG committee of physicians and Ph.D.s. Within a year, the NSGC committee published what is now the standard definition of genetic counseling (see Chapter 3 for details). With their own definition of genetic counseling, the genetic counseling profession took ownership of the clinical practice of genetic counseling. Any attempts to measure the success, conduct, and outcomes of genetic counseling must in some way refer back to this definition.

REFERENCES

Biesecker, B. B., C. W. Vockley, and E. Conover. 1993. "Implications of Human Genome Research: Impact on Graduate Education in Genetic Counseling." *Journal of Genetic Counseling* 2: 213–29.

Carter, C. O. 1967. *Comments on Genetic Counseling*. Proceedings of the 3rd International Conference of Human Genetics, London, England, 97–101.

Comfort, N. 2012. *The Science of Human Perfection*. New Haven, CT: Yale University Press.

Dice, L. R. 1952. "Heredity Clinics: Their Value for Public Service and Research." *American Journal of Human Genetics* 4, no. 1: 1–13.

Emery, A. 1984. *Psychological Aspects of Genetic Counselling*. London: Academic Press.

Eunpu, D. 1997. "Systemically-Based Psychotherapeutic Techniques in Genetic Counseling." *Journal of Genetic Counseling* 6: 1–20.

Evans, C., and P. Harper. 2006. *Genetic Counselling: A Psychological Approach*. Cambridge: Cambridge University Press.

Fiddler, M. B., B. A. Fine, D. L. Baker, ABGC Consensus Development Consortium. 1996. "A Case-Based Approach to the Development of Practice-Based Competencies for Accreditation of and Training in Graduate Programs in Genetic Counseling." *Journal of Genetic Counseling* 5: 105–12. https://doi.org/10.1007/BF01408655

Fine, B. A., D. L. Baker, M. B. Fiddler, ABGC Consensus Development Consortium. 1996. "Practice-Based Competencies for Accreditation of and Training in Graduate Programs in Genetic Counseling." *Journal of Genetic Counseling* 5: 113–21. https://doi.org/10.1007/BF01408656

Fraser Roberts, J. A. 1940. *An Introduction to Medical Genetics*. London: Oxford University Press.

Gorlin, R., and J. Pendborg. 1964. *Syndromes of the Head and Neck*. New York: McGraw Hill.

Griffin, M. L., C. M. Kavanagh, and J. R. Sorenson. 1976–77. "Genetic Knowledge, Client Perspectives, and Genetic Counseling." *Social Work in Health Care* 2, no. 2: 171–80.

Harper, P. 2008. *A Short History of Medical Genetics*. Oxford: Oxford University Press.

Heimler, A. 1997. "An Oral History of the National Society of Genetic Counselors." *Journal of Genetic Counseling* 6: 315–336.

Herndon, C. N. 1955. "Heredity Counseling." *Eugenics Quarterly* 2: 83–89.

Kenen, R. H. 1984. "Genetic counseling: the development of a new interdisciplinary occupational field." *Social Science and Medicine* 18: 541–549.

Kevles, D. J. 1995. *In The Name of Eugenics: Genetics and the Uses of Human Heredity*. 2nd ed. Cambridge, MA: Harvard University Press.

Lindee, S. 2016. "Human genetics after the bomb: Archives, clinics, proving grounds and board rooms." *Studies in History and Philosophy of Biological and Biomedical Sciences* 55: 45–53.

Löwy, I. 2017. *Imperfect Pregnancies—A History of Birth Defects and Prenatal Diagnosis.* Baltimore, MD: Johns Hopkins University Press.

Marks J. 1993. "The Training of Genetic Counselors: Origins of a Psychosocial Model: Ethical Challenges and Consequences." *Prescribing Our Future: Ethical Challenges in Genetic Counseling.* Dianne M. Bartels, Bonnie S. LeRoy, and Arthur L. Caplan, editors. Aldine de Gmyter, Hawthorne, NY, 15–24.

Marks JH, Richter ML. 1976. "The GeneticAssociate: A New Health Professional." *American Journal of Public Health* 66: 388–390.

Paul, D. B. 1995. *Controlling Human Heredity: 1865 to the Present.* Amherst, NY: Humanities Books.

Paul, D. B. 1998. *The Politics of Heredity: Essays on Eugenics, Biomedicine, and the Nature–Nurture Debate.* Albany: State University of New York Press.

Pearson, K. 1912. *The Treasury of Human Inheritance.* London: University of London, Francis Galton Laboratory for National Eugenics.

Reed, S. J. 1955. *Counseling in Medical Genetics.* Philadelphia: WB Saunders.

Resta, R. G., ed. 2000. *Psyche and Helix—Psychological Aspects of Genetic Counseling, Essays by Seymour Kessler, Ph.D.* New York: Wiley-Liss.

Resta, R. 2010. "The Great Genetic Counseling Divorce of 1992." https://thednaexchange.com/2010/04/11/the-great-genetic-counseling-divorce-of-1992-a-historical-perspective-on-change-in-the-genetic-counseling-profession/, accessed June 16, 2018.

Schild, S., and R. Beck Black. 1984. *Social Work and Genetics—A Guide for Practice.* New York: Haworth Press.

Smith, D. W. 1970. *Recognizable Patterns of Human Malformation.* Philadelphia: WB Saunders.

Snyder, L. H. 1941. *Medical Genetics: A Series of Lectures Presented to the Medical Schools of Duke University, Wake Forest College, and the University of North Carolina.* Durham, NC: Duke University Press.

Stern, A. M. 2012. *Telling Genes—The Story of Genetic Counseling in America.* Baltimore, MD: Johns Hopkins University Press.

Targum, S. D. 1981. "Psychotherapeutic Considerations in Genetic Counseling." *American Journal of Medical Genetics* 8: 281–89.

Walker, A. 1998. "The Practice of Genetic Counseling." in *A Guide to Genetic Counseling.* Baker D, Schuette J, Uhlmann W. 1st Edition. Wiley-Liss, NY, 1–26.

Walker, A. P., Scott, J. A., Biesecker, B. B., Conover, B. 1990. "Report of the 1989 Asilomar meeting on education in genetic counseling." *American Journal of Human Genetics* 46: 1223–1230.

Warkany, J. 1971. *Congenital Malformations. Notes and Comments.* Chicago: Year Book Medical.

Weil, J. 2000. *Psychosocial Genetic Counseling.* New York: Oxford University Press.

CHAPTER 3

Definitions and Goals of Genetic Counseling

To begin a description of the definitions and goals of counseling, we reflect on our model of genetic counseling, one that we originally described as psychoeducational and more recently as psychotherapeutic (Biesecker, Austin, and Caleshu 2017a, 2017b; Biesecker and Peters 2001). In the most literal sense, the first descriptor, psychoeducational, is a better fit and appears more often in the literature. It encapsulates both the teaching and counseling paradigms of genetic counseling that Dr. Seymour Kessler differentiated, each with its distinct goals (Kessler 1997). This psychoeducational model recognizes that often clients are seeking information and that the information has both affective and cognitive consequences. We have evolved in our thinking to promote a psychotherapeutic model of genetic counseling (Biesecker et al. 2017a, 2017b) in concordance with Jehannine Austin's argument that genetic counseling shares characteristics with psychotherapy (Austin et al. 2014).

Genetic counseling is often described in the media as a public resource for obtaining useful information on interpretation of heritable risk from genetic testing. Box 3.1 is the description of genetic counseling offered by the Centers for Disease Control and Prevention (CDC). As such, genetic counseling appears to be taking on an identity as an information service rather than a psychotherapeutic process. Evidence discussed throughout this text echoes concerns about genetic counseling that were raised in the early years of the profession by Dr. Kessler (1979). That is, if the practice of genetic counseling favors an educational or informational service model, it is at a cost to our clients.

> **Text Box 3.1**
> **CDC DESCRIPTION OF GENETIC COUNSELING**
>
> Genetic counseling gives you information about how genetic conditions might affect you or your family. The genetic counselor or other healthcare professional will collect your personal and family health history. They can use this information to determine how likely it is that you or your family member has a genetic condition. Based on this information, the genetic counselor can help you decide whether a genetic test might be right for you or your relative (https://www.cdc.gov/genomics/gtesting/genetic_counseling.htm.)

Evidence of practice (Meiser et al. 2008) and public perceptions have obscured the role of genetic counseling in addressing the psychological impact of genetics—specifically, how the threat of a health risk or the diagnosis of a condition is processed by a client and elicits affective and cognitive responses that shape how the information is understood, acted on, and shared with others at risk. These patient-related outcomes are central to determining the effectiveness of genetic counseling and illustrate the importance of a psychotherapeutic counseling model to guide genetic counselors as they help clients and families manage their responses to genetic information. This model we describe in detail in Chapter 8.

Accordingly, a practice model depends on the definition of practice. As you will see in this chapter, historical definitions of genetic counseling follow the evolution of genetic counseling practice from its origins in the prevention of birth defects, to information communication, to the integration of education and psychotherapeutic counseling. Remarkably, only fairly recently have US genetic counselors been consistent in describing what they aim to accomplish in their clinical practice. The National Society of Genetic Counselors has prioritized identification of client and patient outcomes that are most highly sought and valued (https://www.nsgc.org/page/nsgc-outcomes-measure-developer-rfp).

An initial educational practice model likely arose from geneticists' enthusiasm about emerging clinical information that could be offered to patients for understanding of genetic diagnoses and inheritance (Stevenson and Davison 1970). It would have been consistent with parents' and patients' expressed desires to understand the condition in their child or family. Yet a primarily educational model, referred to by Dr. Kessler as the "teaching model of genetic counseling," falls short in addressing clients' broad responses to the information (Kessler 1997).

Many assumptions belie a strictly educational model about the primary importance of genetic information in managing risk or informing reproductive decisions. The assumptions include high regard for the primacy of information and reinforce the notion that knowledge breeds control and mastery over risk. It follows that provision of accurate genetic information allows clients the opportunity to make not only informed choices but also rational decisions that are more closely aligned with the decision outcomes valued by genetics providers. It assumes that less rational decisions are misinformed or based on genetic ignorance, while they may actually be informed and based on patient preferences. When the context is preference-based decision making, an informed choice is the objective.*

A psychoeducational model (Biesecker and Peters 2001; Resta et al. 2006) embraces the affective and cognitive responses to genetic information that influence interpretation and meaning. Dr. Abby Lippman interviewed women who had undergone prenatal genetic counseling about the meaning they made of the information (Lippman-Hand and Fraser 1979b, 1979a, 1979d, 1979c). Lippman demonstrated that many women's mental model for fetal risk was 50/50: it was either going to happen or not. Interestingly, Dr. Lippman's findings illustrate a heuristic, a cognitive shortcut, often used to make personal meaning of probabilistic information (Tversky and Kahneman 1974). You may have experienced clients using this heuristic, most notably when they remark on their risk, "So it's either going to happen or not, right?"

Clients who learn of an increased genetic risk or a diagnosis and appraise it as a significant threat to their health may experience psychological distress (Meiser and Quinn 2018), lower quality of life (Umstead et al. 2018), social stigmatization (Kumar et al. 2019), and changes to their self-identity (Berkenstadt et al. 1999; Fanos 1999a, 1999b; Fanos et al. 2011; Kessler 1979; Lippman-Hand and Fraser 1979b). Yet despite the potential for these outcomes, clients most often benefit from genetic information. Receiving accurate information can lead to patient relief from cognitive and affective uncertainties (Han et al. 2017) and gains in empowerment (McAllister and Dearing 2015) and can leave clients better equipped to make informed choices (Dormandy, Tsui, and Marteau 2007; Marteau, Dormandy, and Crockett 2005). The degree to which clients have negative affective responses varies by how psychologically and medically threatening the information is.

At a minimum, the information provided by genetic counselors is likely to leave clients feeling somewhat vulnerable. Affective responses can be influenced by clients' background, needs, and expectations for genetic counseling (Peters and Petrill 2011a, 2011b). Prior personal experiences

---

* This does not pertain to making health behavior recommendations. These are medically indicated and are not preference-based decisions.

with the condition or risk in the family generate perceptions of the degree of burden of the condition and personal loss that are key determinants of the psychological perceived impact of the information (Lippman-Hand and Fraser 1979b).

Notably, those with experience with the condition may perceive less threat as they have seen their relatives mount the challenges. Among affected families, predictive risk information may be perceived as empowering and a source for at-risk relatives to make informed choices (Bell 2012; Caswell-Jin, Zimmer, and Stedden 2019; Cheung et al. 2010; Elrick et al. 2017). Appreciating the context in which the information is delivered to clients can reveal the individualized and personal nature of genetic information. Effective genetic counseling respects clients' prior experience with a genetic condition or risk, while exploring responses that may emerge from learning novel or unexpected information.

PRACTICE DEFINITIONS

Over its relatively short history as a professional practice, genetic counseling has been defined several ways. The first practice definitions originated in North America and were not explicitly distinct from the aim of preventing birth defects. These origins raised questions about the initial intent of genetic counseling and periodically continue to raise concerns about how successfully genetic counseling has evolved beyond them (Duster 1990). In her seminal history of genetic counseling, Dr. Alexandra Stern (2012) includes a memo written in 1968 by Dr. Melissa Richter, who established the first genetic counseling program at Sarah Lawrence College. In the memo, Dr. Richter described the intent of a "new health counseling service" to be the prevention of birth defects. Although the descriptor that rapidly gained favor was "nondirective," aimed at declaring that the practice upheld autonomous decision making to act on genetic risk information, a shadow was cast over the goals of genetic counseling.[†]

In the foreword to Kessler's textbook, *Genetic Counseling: Psychological Dimensions*, Epstein reviews several early practice definitions, each of which includes a goal to prevent or reduce the incidence of birth defects (Kessler 1979). By 1979, these definitions emphasized communicating genetic information and helping clients make decisions. Epstein comments on the notable switch in emphasis from prevention to counseling; however, somewhat paradoxically, he later remarks that prevention of birth defects

---

[†] The original source that introduced nondirectiveness into the profession is uncertain.

remained a goal of genetic counseling (Kessler 1979). If we reflect back, perhaps by "prevention of birth defects" Epstein meant offering reproductive choices when fetuses were affected with a birth defect. Epstein may also have been referring to arming parents with information about heritable risks so they could make informed reproductive decisions prior to pregnancy. Regardless, the goal of preventing birth defects is reminiscent of eugenic intent and a reminder that the options offered to clients and patients in genetic counseling may be interpreted by some as efforts to avoid the birth of affected fetuses.

In the late 1970s, families affected by genetic conditions were speaking out to the medical genetics community to convey that they were not uniformly interested in preventing the condition in their family. About this time, scientists and others declared that the prevention of all birth defects and genetic conditions was unattainable due to the rate of spontaneous mutations in the population and the largely unknown, and thereby unalterable, cause of many birth defects. While scientists vocalized the unrealistic nature of the prevention goal, it remained in the shadows of genetic counseling. Dr. Troy Duster (1990) discusses the complexities of prevention in genetic counseling, including disparities in access to services, in his insightful book *Backdoor to Eugenics* (Duster 1990). Undoubtedly, there is a fine line between informed reproductive choices and prevention of the birth of affected children. On that line straddles the opportunity for parents to make autonomous decisions in line with their values, beliefs, and resources.

Almost everyone embarking on a pregnancy aims to have a baby unaffected by a structural or developmental abnormality. At present, prevention of birth defects is not limited to termination of affected pregnancies. Rubella vaccination is given to prevent fetal rubella syndrome. Folic acid is recommended to women planning a pregnancy to prevent neural tube defects. It is probably fair to say that most women, even the most ardent supporters of people with disabilities, would choose to have the rubella vaccination and take folic acid. Yet, the assumption that if clients are given accurate information on the genetic cause of a condition in their family, they will use the information to avoid the birth of future affected children suggests to some that the lives of those affected are less worthy (Parens and Asch 2003). This implication results in tensions between the views and priorities of disability advocates and genetic counselors, and greater tensions around reproductive rights in the United States (Dent et al. 2011; Madeo et al. 2011).

While parents armed with accurate genetic information may be presumed to make "good" decisions that result in the birth of fewer affected children, families with affected relatives espouse the virtues of living in a diverse society. A vocal majority claims that greater sensibilities, appreciation, and grace emanate from the value of the lives of their affected relatives (Parens and Asch 2000). While this seems to be the consensus view among advocates, the perspective of parents who have fewer resources to raise and care for a child with a developmental or medical challenge may not be fully represented in these views and may differ. Further, these parents may have fewer opportunities to access prenatal testing to make informed decisions for their families.

When clients make an informed choice that is based on sufficient understanding of the genetics information provided and that is in line with their attitudes (determined by personal values and beliefs), the collective outcome may be perceived (globally) as occurring in the interest of maintaining the "health" of the population. As such, genetic counseling has long grappled with a subtle or unspoken goal of preventing genetic conditions, even after the goal was eliminated from practice definitions. Providers find comfort in upholding the goal of prevention if it is actualized by clients using their free will to make autonomous informed decisions to terminate affected pregnancies. This may be broadly recognized as a covert, though not deliberate, effort to prevent birth defects in a morally acceptable way (Duster 1990).

Genetic counseling continues to generate tensions around the reduction of the incidence of people affected with genetic conditions or birth defects as remarkable advances in technology are occurring. Treatment and prevention of rare diseases through application of expanding technologies, such as CRISPR (Clustered Regularly Interspaced Short Palindromic Repeats), predict healthier futures for those affected with genetic conditions. Examples include a recent announcement about individuals cured of sickle cell disease (https://sicklecellanemianews.com/2018/05/08/stem-cells-from-half-matched-donors-cure-sickle-cell-adult-patients-study-reports/).

While providing hope for patients and parents of affected children, this progress exacerbates the complications of how to consider the value of living life affected by a genetic condition. An overarching human goal is to prevent disease and suffering, so improved treatments and prevention are nearly universally welcomed; yet respect for human differences and inclusion of those with disabilities in our society is also a strong value upheld by most, and particularly by many genetic counselors (see Chapter 5 for discussion of genetic counselors' values).

Following emphasis on prevention were practice definitions about communication. In North America, a commonly cited definition of genetic counseling for many years was written in 1974 by a committee of the American Society of Human Genetics (ASHG), chaired by Dr, Clarke

Fraser. This definition has several components but focuses primarily on the communication process between family and counselor:

> Genetic counseling is a communication process which deals with the human problems associated with the occurrence or risk of occurrence of a genetic disorder in a family. This process involves an attempt by one or more appropriately trained persons to help the individual or family to: (1) comprehend the medical facts including the diagnosis, probable course of the disorder, and the available management, (2) appreciate the way heredity contributes to the disorder and the risk of recurrence in specified relatives, (3) understand the alternatives for dealing with the risk of recurrence, (4) choose a course of action which seems to them appropriate in view of their risk, their family goals, and their ethical and religious standards and act in accordance with that decision, and (5) to make the best possible adjustment to the disorder in an affected family member and/or to the risk of recurrence of that disorder. (Fraser 1974, p. 637)

Although others have declared that the ASHG practice definition remained relevant for twenty-five years (Walker 1998), two of us argued that the field of genetic counseling had evolved sufficiently by the early twenty-first century to warrant a more contemporary practice definition (Biesecker and Peters 2001). Genetic counseling, while often practiced in conjunction with medical genetics, is a distinct certified profession. In the United States, specialization of genetic counseling in oncology, cardiology, neurology, and ophthalmology means that genetic counselors often work within clinical teams where they function as the genetics expert without the presence of medical geneticists. Clear differentiation of genetic counseling from genetic diagnosis and medical management is important in distinguishing the roles of medical practitioners from those of genetic counselors. The accuracy of a diagnosis is critically important to informing the genetic information provided to clients, yet making the diagnosis is the purview of medical genetics and distinct from the expertise of genetic counselors. Yet even this paradigm has shifted through the use of genetic testing. Many diagnoses and risks can be verified by a test result that is interpreted by a genetic counselor.

Genetic counseling has been described in the professional literature as a series of tasks. In 1994, the American Board of Genetic Counseling (ABGC) convened a consensus development conference to identify a core set of practice-based competencies (Fine, Baker, and Fiddler 1996; Fiddler et al. 1996). Using a case-based narrative method, genetic counseling graduate program directors, education and accreditation consultants, and the ABGC board of directors together drafted genetic counselor competencies. They included:

> a) eliciting and interpreting individual and family medical, developmental, and reproductive histories; b) determining the mode of inheritance and risk of occurrence and

recurrence of genetic conditions and birth defects; c) explaining the etiology, natural history, diagnosis, and management of these conditions; d) interpreting and explaining the results of genetic tests and other diagnostic studies; e) performing a psychosocial assessment to identify emotional, social, educational, and cultural issues; f) evaluating the client's and/or family's responses to the condition or risk of occurrence; g) providing client-centered counseling and anticipatory guidance; h) promoting informed decision-making about testing, management, reproduction, and communication with family members; i) identifying and using community resources that provide medical, educational, financial, and psychosocial support and advocacy; and j) providing written documentation of medical, genetic, and counseling information for families and other health professionals. (Fine et al. 1996)

In 1996, the ABGC endorsed these competencies (Fine et al. 1996; Fiddler et al. 1996). They served as a basis for professional certification and graduate program accreditation in the United States. Both were critical achievements in the professional development of master's-trained genetic counselors. Although there is a paucity of empirical evidence to support these competencies as critical to practice, their delineation has importantly contributed to standardization of genetic counseling training and likely to genetic counseling practice. Certification and accreditation served as cornerstones to the specifications of how genetic counselors should be trained and what level of achievement was considered necessary to meet clients' needs.

Three central components of genetic counseling (to teach, counsel, and advocate) are suggested by the competencies. Yet, the competencies were determined without context. They generally fail to include assessment of client needs or how these skills are to be used to meet genetic counseling goals. The purpose served by the information, whether it is aimed at what the client seeks to learn or what the expectations are for clients to act on the information, is unstated. These early competencies were derived from counselors' perspectives of what they ought to be sharing with their clients. As such, they are not client-centered outcomes (even if they do serve clients), they are not evidence-based (because no evidence existed), and they originated from a small group of professional leaders. Regardless of these limitations, these original competencies served to instigate standardization for training and practice.

Given the limitations of prior definitions, practice competencies, and the evolving practice of genetic counseling, two of us proposed a novel practice definition in 2001 with explicit practice goals (Biesecker and Peters 2001):

Genetic counseling is a dynamic *psychoeducational* process centered on genetic information. Within a therapeutic relationship established between providers and clients,

clients are helped to personalize technical and probabilistic genetic information, to promote self-determinism and to enhance their ability to adapt over time. The goal is to facilitate clients' ability to use genetic information in a personally meaningful way that minimizes psychological distress and increases personal control. (p. 194)

This definition describes genetic counseling provided by trained experts working with diverse patients in any clinical setting. Specialization in genetic counseling makes it increasingly challenging to define the practice in a way that unifies the many facets of the profession. Yet, it is this very diversity within genetic counseling that makes it increasingly important for there to be a central definition of the practice and stated goals. This definition emphasizes the therapeutic relationship that facilitates exploration of the meaning of and succeeding adaption to the genetic information for the client. Our proposed definition was a departure from prior emphases on diagnosis, communication, and, more subtly, prevention. In keeping with the discourse of reproductive ethics, the definition upholds respect for self-determinism (Wertz and Gregg 2002) and embraces the education and counseling components. It rests on the theoretical and empirical evidence for the adaptation process people progress through when encountering a personal health threat (Kessler 1979; Taylor 1983). It contributed to the literature on practice definitions and may have informed the 2003 decision by the National Society of Genetic Counselors (NSGC) to appoint a task force to create a practice definition for the profession.

Two of us (Resta and Biesecker) participated in the 2005 NSGC task force (Resta et al. 2006). We reviewed past practice definitions, assessed their limitations, considered the rising variety of subspecialty practices, and determined the need to create a definition that applied generically to all settings. Care was taken to differentiate genetic counseling practice as distinct from tasks conducted by genetic counselors. The latter were recognized to be important but more context-specific and represented by ABGC practice competencies and thus more relevant to graduate training in genetic counseling than to practicing professionals. The task force found it challenging to differentiate the essence of the practice from the skills and activities undertaken by genetic counselors in practice. The definition was intended to be universal to context, setting, provider, and location across North America, yet it is unknown how well it represents genetic counseling practice worldwide. The following is the definition resulting from the NSGC committee's efforts:

Genetic counseling is the process of helping people understand and adapt to the medical, psychological, and familial implications of genetic contributions to disease. This process integrates:

- Interpretation of family and medical histories to assess the chance of disease occurrence or recurrence
- Education about inheritance, testing, management, prevention, resources, and research
- Counseling to promote informed choices and adaptation to the risk or condition. (Resta et al., 2006, p. 77)

In 2018, the authors of this 2006 definition informally reconvened to assess whether it remained relevant twelve years hence, in light of the remarkable expansion of professional roles (Resta et al. 2006). We sought to assess how frequently the definition has been cited, and whether and how it is taught in graduate programs across the United States and beyond. An informal survey of program directors found that ten international training programs use the 2006 definition as a reference point throughout training. Typically, it is shared with students early in their training and contrasted to country-specific sociocultural differences, which may be covered by the definition but actualized differently in practice. As of May 4, 2018, the definition was cited in sixty-one references in PubMed Central, 465 references in Google Scholar, 342 references in ResearchGate, and 276 references in CrossRef. In the *Journal of Genetic Counseling*, the definition article was in the ninety-ninth percentile for citations. The relevance of the definition seems to be holding up well in the United States and overseas, which our author group found to be quite validating of its continued relevance. We do advocate for the importance of periodically revisiting the definition to reassess its appropriateness in light of practice advances.

GOALS OF GENETIC COUNSELING

Practice goals emerge from the model and the definition of genetic counseling. In keeping with the NSGC definition and our proposed model, the primary goals of genetic counseling resemble those of other psychoeducational counseling interactions: promoting understanding, facilitating decision making, achieving client informed choice, reducing psychological distress, enhancing perceptions of personal control, and advancing adaptation to health-threatening information and experiences (Resta et al. 2006). These client-centered objectives represent an expanded view of genetic counseling practice, which initially placed emphasis on the communication of genetic information to inform decision making.

Responses and behaviors of genetic counseling clients are not unique but rather follow the common course of psychological processes of individuals experiencing stressful life events. Genetic counseling practice recognizes that clients generally have inner strength to appraise and cope with genetic risk or a genetic condition in their family with time. Yet their initial responses are the need to make meaning of the health threat and align their resources for coping with the stress it generates (Taylor 1983). Genetic counselors have potent opportunities to assist in the process of psychological adaptation to genetic information (Biesecker and Erby 2008).

When clients first learn genetic information, the counselor focuses on helping them begin the process of making meaning of the information. If it is unexpected, a shock response is expected: The clients are taking in what they can but will benefit from compassionate regard above all else. After the clients have absorbed the implications of the information, the goal of genetic counseling is to help them appraise the degree of health threat and identify their resources, such as opportunities for taking control and gaining confidence in their ability to cope. Later, after time has passed since the information was learned, the goal of genetic counseling is enhancing clients' coping abilities, with the longer-term objective of adapting to the condition or risk. Missing an opportunity to help clients assimilate difficult information is to skirt our professional responsibilities to our clients and, worse, our moral obligations to one another as compassionate fellow human beings.

It is expected that clients will need time to adapt, and the time they need depends in large measure on the degree of threat posed. For example, if the diagnosis of a genetic condition, such as Cornelia de Lange, confirms unexplained concerns a couple has had about their baby, the diagnosis may provide some relief and valuable information for a couple striving to make sense of their concerns about their child. In contrast, if there is no prior awareness of a problem or concern, a diagnosis of Cornelia de Lange will likely come as a shock and the couple would be reeling from the information—barely able to comprehend what was being said to them. Recognizing the circumstances and likely state of mind of clients is important so that the counselor can engage with them effectively. A counselor may choose to acknowledge to parents that while it is a terribly painful process, most people adapt over time. This may provide a kernel of hope for the future in what may feel like a hopeless circumstance. Yet if this comment is made just as the parents are learning that something is significantly different with their child, this comment would be of little help and may even hurt the parents. You can imagine them thinking, "We are not 'most people'!" "What if we don't adapt?" Genetic counselors need to have a clear understanding of the state of psychological well-being of their clients. If the parents have had time to absorb the circumstances, counselors can reinforce their role by being available to help the family through a challenging time and offer great comfort to the parents. Timing in the delivery of further information or counseling interventions is critical to their effectiveness, and hinge on empathic understanding of one's clients.

It is insufficient to describe the goal of genetic counseling as being "supportive." This term is vague and, when offered to clients, can leave them feeling unmoored. It may also conflict with what clients expect from the genetic counseling encounter (Peters and Petrill 2011a, 2011b). What does it mean to tell our clients that we "support them at this difficult time" or "support whatever decision they make"? While well intended, these phrases represent a form of emotional disengagement. Further, such statements can be confusing for clients, who in general look to clinical providers to take on the role of responsible decision makers in medical situations.

Genetic counseling demands more than a vague notion of offering support. It involves establishing an active partnership with a client to a degree where the counselor takes risks to connect with the client on an personal level. To help a parent make an informed choice, the counselor ensures that the client understands the information, is acting in accordance with his or her values and beliefs, and makes a decision that is consistent and psychologically sound given the circumstances and context of his or her life. One challenging circumstance in genetic counseling that can arise is that parents often hold themselves responsible for their child's condition and may hang on to a particular explanation (causal attribution) because it serves an important psychological function. For example, if a mother believes it was the bathroom cleaner she used during her pregnancy that led to her baby's condition, the causative agent may be avoided in future pregnancies. This attribution, while almost certainly inaccurate, provides a way for her to perceive that she has control over the health of her future children, and it may prove particularly important to her psychological well-being should she have more children. The good news for counselors eager to disabuse her of her erroneous attribution is that evidence finds that maintaining an explanation such as the bathroom cleaner does not seem to impede accepting that the child has a genetic condition. Most parents (and patients) are capable of holding multiple causal attributions to explain their child's condition (Dong et al. 2005) A common example is to believe that a condition was God's will and resulted from chromosomal nondisjunction. One of these attributions does not exclude the other; rather, they work together to give a parent a reason and meaning for the child's genetic status. As such, a goal of genetic counseling should be to uphold causal attributions that parents (and patients) assign to their child's condition without disabusing them of their causal role, while supplying a scientific attribution that can be simultaneously accepted. It serves no useful purpose for a genetic counselor to try to convince parents that the scientific attribution is the only explanation.

Failing to engage clients in a therapeutic encounter can happen rather innocently if the counselor tries to reassure parents after a diagnosis has been made that the child is "the same child that walked in the door an hour earlier" and that nothing has changed beyond placing a label on the child's characteristics. This is commonly told to parents who have engaged in a journey to arrive at a diagnosis. But this message—that things are "just the same"—likely differs substantially from the parents' viewpoint. From the perspective of the family, they have replaced general uncertainty about their child's condition with specific uncertainty about how a condition will manifest, the risks to others in the family, and how to share this information with family members and friends. Yet, the uncertain, but "open," future for their child, entails limited parameters on how the child's life may unfold and so also often gives yield to hope. Receiving a diagnosis can bring relief and more certainty, but it also likely means that going forward will be quite different for the child and family. Providing reassuring platitudes often serve the provider by making him or her more comfortable in the face of delivering a diagnosis rather than addressing clients' needs. It is only when we engage with clients in an empathic relationship that we can begin to understand what a diagnosis means to them and not try to take that meaning away but to understand it, even when we might not consider it to be scientific or fully rational.

Our clients' perceptions are personal and important to their well-being and that of their family. An aim within the process of genetic counseling is to understand the implications of the genetic information from the clients' perspective rather than attempting to persuade them to accept our scientific and/or psychological view. Clients make their own meaning of the information. We need to avoid trying to normalize or minimize the fears and concerns that accompany learning a diagnosis. While genetic counseling aims to convey accurate and relevant genetic information to clients, it needs to be personalized in the context of their existing cognitive and affective needs.

Most genetic counseling clients are psychologically healthy and have the personal resources to withstand the impact of learning health-threatening information about themselves or their relatives. The professional literature on coping with chronic illness suggests that people are stressed to learn they are at increased health risk but that, over time, they find ways to adapt, even when the circumstances are grave (Lazarus and Folkman 1984). It is important to remember that, generally, adults and children adapt to health threats on their own, often without the assistance of health care providers. Clients tend to rely on family, social networks, and personal resources, not just those offered by the medical profession. Increasingly, the internet offers online support and advocacy groups to connect with other patients and parents of children with the same condition, even among parents whose child is undiagnosed. These connections, whether informal or formalized in advocacy organizations, can provide parents with relevant, condition-specific information and suggestions of ways to cope with the threat of the condition to their child.

Shelley Taylor (1983) posited a theory of adaptation that has been supported by evidence into sustaining threats or injuries, including cancer, rape, and heart disease. Evidence supports that clients progress through three dimensions of the adaptation process in response to a threat: (1) a search for meaning in the experience, (2) an attempt to regain mastery over the event in particular and over one's life in general, and (3) an effort to enhance one's self-esteem—that is, to feel good about oneself again despite the setback. The majority of people facing illness or loss achieve a quality of life or level of happiness equivalent to or even exceeding their prior level of satisfaction (Andreasen and Norris 1972; Katz 1963; Myers, Friedman, and Weiner 1970; Tavormina et al. 1976; Visotsky 1961; Weisman and Sobel 1979; Wortman and Silver 1989). The prevalence of client adaptation to genetic conditions, based on measures of quality of life and psychological well-being, is notably high (Athens et al. 2017; Cohen and Biesecker 2010; Sulzer et al. 1962).

Evidence supports an existential view of clients as remarkably capable and inherently adaptive (Biesecker et al. 2013; Cohen and Biesecker 2010; Sutton et al. 2006; Turriff, Levy, and Biesecker 2015). While such a view provides health care providers with a dynamic framework for assessing client reactions to health-threatening information, this is not to say that all clients adapt in the same way, or that some clients do not suffer considerably during the process. It may be lengthy and particularly difficult for some clients. They may experience depressive symptoms, isolation, social stigma, and adverse effects on family relationships (Biesecker et al. 2013; Gray et al. 2017; Green et al. 2001). There are many opportunities for counselors to employ interventions to enhance the adaptation process (see Chapter 8).

Genetic counseling that focuses primarily on providing information and answering clients' questions would be enhanced by understanding the broad context in which the questions are being asked, such as Taylor's cognitive adaptation theory (1983). Educational efforts are significantly more effective if they are made personally relevant to the client and are tailored to fit the client's needs. In this way, they interdigitate with engagement in a therapeutic relationship. A psychoeducational approach tailors not only the information but also the counseling approach. A couple who has suspected a problem in their baby for some time may be ready to incorporate new information and to process what it may mean not only for the baby but also for themselves. They may be prepared to discuss how frightening it has been to realize that something so substantial is wrong with their infant and how scared and isolated they have been feeling. Acknowledging these feelings in a meaningful way may be the important start of an empathic connection. These feelings do not likely to dissipate rapidly, and it can be a powerful experience for parents to discuss them and to feel "heard." Yet none of us outside of their experience can truly understand. This is the nature of empathy; we understand as if it were us, but without ever neglecting the "as if" circumstance.

A unifying practice model and definition will not lead directly to singularity in practice goals as they vary by setting and client needs. Goals are less about what the genetic counselor thinks that clients need and more about what the clients think and feel they need. To practice client-centered care, genetic counselors need to consider their clients' beliefs, values, understanding, relevant experiences, and preferences. When these clash with the priorities of counselors or are based on misinformation, a patient-centered negotiation of the goals may be needed, although this is not essential if the clients assess that their goals have been met. Specific practice goals (Biesecker 2001) by subspecialty follow.

Prenatal genetic counseling aims to help clients make informed choices as such; the goal is *to promote clients' self-determination in exercising reproductive choices*. The specific aims of prenatal counseling are (1) delivering personalized genomic information to clients in a meaningful way; (2) partnering with clients to explore the meaning of the information in the context of their personal values and beliefs; (3) promoting clients' preferences for reproductive options with consideration of alternatives, consequences, and barriers; and (4) preparing clients for accepting the consequences of their decision.

In the majority of cases presenting to a pediatric or adult genetics clinic, a family member is affected with a condition and the patient or parents are seeking to learn the diagnosis, prognosis, and recurrence risks. As such, the goal is *to facilitate client understanding, meaning making, appraisals, coping, and adaptation*. The specific aims of pediatric/adult genetic counseling are (1) exploring clients' understanding of the cause; (2) promoting feelings of mastery over a condition and appraisals of one's abilities to manage it; and (3) enhancing coping effectiveness to facilitate adaptation to the condition.

Genetic counseling in oncology, neurology, cardiology, ophthalmology, and psychiatry addresses risk for more common complex genetic disease and options for predictive testing. The goals of genetic counseling for common diseases are *to understand personalized disease risk and to enhance health-promoting behaviors*. The specific aims of genetic counseling for common diseases are (1) enhancing accuracy of risk perceptions; (2) promoting health-enhancing behaviors; (3) facilitating adaptation to genetic risk; and (4) detecting disease early and/or preventing it.

PRACTICE OUTCOMES

The application of practice definitions, such as the NSGC 2006 definition, and the above-stated goals, need to be studied to assess their appropriateness and usefulness to client care. To pursue this line of research, some consensus on key client outcomes of genetic counseling is needed. In psychotherapy, outcome studies often focus on observable client changes such as improved psychological well-being, satisfaction, problem-solving, social adaptation, reduction of negative symptoms (such as distress or anxiety), or behavior change. Some of these outcomes have been assessed in genetic counseling studies designed by investigators trained in health behavior, and health or social psychology (Chapter 10).

Genetic counseling outcome studies have sought to assess how well the process worked to educate the client (Meiser et al., 2008), satisfy the client, or facilitate decision making (reproductive or test decisions) (Evers-Kiebooms and van den Berghe 1979; Michie, Marteau, and Bobrow 1997; Michie, McDonald, and Marteau, 1997; Shiloh, Avdor, and Goodman 1990; Sorenson et al. 1981; Wertz and Fletcher 1988). An exploratory study of genetic counselors and a sample of their clients argued for outcomes that included the client's sense of being heard, encouraged, valued, and attended to as well as improved family communication, anticipation of future feelings and experiences, and clarification of personal beliefs and values shaping decisions and attitudes (Bernhardt, Biesecker, and Mastromarino 2000).

Many of these "outcomes" instead relate to the process of genetic counseling where clients can have a voice and are respected by the genetic counselor. These processes, described in detail in Chapter 8, are key to establishing a therapeutic relationship and pave the way for positive client outcomes. To train genetic counselors, findings from process studies can be very useful, particularly when they are linked to desirable outcomes. To assess the effectiveness of genetic counseling, we need to further investigate what aspects of counseling our clients believed was beneficial to them.

In the 2010s, focus groups of genetic counselors held at sequential NSGC conferences were conducted to assess perceptioms of practice outcomes (Redlinger-Grosse et al. 2016; Zerhuit et al. 2016). Using the proposed domains of the Reciprocal Engagement Model (Veach, Bartels, and LeRoy 2007) the findings resulted in the publication of extensive lists of constructs proposed as outcomes (Redlinger-Grosse et al. 2016). Yet many items listed also feature as process variables. While a laudable effort to advance research in genetic counseling, these publications may have obscured what constitutes priorities for assessing practice effectiveness. Ideally research into desired outcomes should be conducted as patient-reported outcomes, rather than outcomes reported by providers. While there can be a role for both, if providers are aiming for different outcomes than their clients, their assessment will not lead to effective practice.

To this end, Dr. Marion McAllister and colleagues (2001) endeavored to assess client-reported outcomes by surveying patients who had received medical genetics services. These efforts resulted in the development of the Genetic Counseling Outcome Scale (GCOS), which has been subsequently validated in several studies. The original scale included twenty-four items, which included "receiving a diagnosis"—this would be a goal of the medical visit, not an outcome to assess genetic counseling. The GCOS has been shortened to six items that are specific to genetic counseling and assess the construct of patient empowerment, called the Genomics Counseling Scale (Grant et al. 2019). These are the only genetic counseling outcome scales based on patient-reported outcomes.

Determining primary outcomes for genetic counseling continues to be a high priority in research (see Chapter 9 for further discussion). A critical aspect of practice outcomes is how well they represent patient needs and reflect the practice model, definition, and goals as presented in this chapter. Of greatest importance are the outcomes of genetic counseling most highly valued by our clients.

SUMMARY

This chapter discusses a general practice model, summarizes definitions of genetic counseling, and proposes practice goals and the need for an array of evidence-based outcomes for assessment. Genetic counseling is psychoeducational in that it recognizes the importance of both genetics information and its impact on the lives of clients. It incorporates the goals of enhancing informed choice and facilitating adaptation to genetic conditions or risk. Such goals lead to client outcomes related to successful psychological adaptation. Assessing the value of genetic counseling for our diverse clients is of great importance to an evolving profession. Later in the text we explore genetic counseling as psychotherapeutic to emphasize the importance of the psychological counseling components of care.

REFERENCES

Andreasen, N. J., and A. S. Norris. 1972. "Long-Term Adjustment and Adaptation Mechanisms in Severely Burned Adults." *Journal of Nervous and Mental Disease* 154, no. 5: 352–62. http://www.ncbi.nlm.nih.gov/pubmed/4260337.

Athens, Barbara A., Samantha L. Caldwell, Kendall L. Umstead, Philip D. Connors, Ethan Brenna, and Barbara B. Biesecker. 2017. "A Systematic Review of Randomized Controlled Trials to Assess Outcomes of Genetic Counseling." *Journal of Genetic Counseling* 26, no. 5: 902–33. https://doi.org/10.1007/s10897-017-0082-y.

Bell, K. 2012. "Exploring Family Communication of BRCA Mutation Results and Uptake of Predictive Genetic Testing in a Clinical Setting." *Current Oncology* 19, no. 2: e109.

Berkenstadt, M., S. Shiloh, G. Barkai, M. B. Katznelson, and B. Goldman. 1999. "Perceived Personal Control (PPC): A New Concept in Measuring Outcome of Genetic Counseling." *American Journal of Medical Genetics* 82, no. 1: 53–59. http://www.ncbi.nlm.nih.gov/pubmed/9916844.

Bernhardt, B. A., B. B. Biesecker, and C. L. Mastromarino. 2000. "Goals, Benefits, and Outcomes of Genetic Counseling: Client and Genetic Counselor Assessment." *American Journal of Medical Genetics* 94, no. 3: 189–97. http://www.ncbi.nlm.nih.gov/pubmed/10995504.

Biesecker, Barbara B. 2001. "Goals of Genetic Counseling." *Clinical Genetics* 60, no. 5: 323–30. http://www.ncbi.nlm.nih.gov/pubmed/11903329.

Biesecker, Barbara, Jehannine Austin, and Colleen Caleshu. 2017a. "Response to a Different Vantage Point Commentary: Psychotherapeutic Genetic Counseling, Is It?" *Journal of Genetic Counseling* 26, no. 2: 334–36. https://doi.org/10.1007/s10897-016-0025-z.

Biesecker, Barbara, Jehannine Austin, and Colleen Caleshu. 2017b. "Theories for Psychotherapeutic Genetic Counseling: Fuzzy Trace Theory and Cognitive Behavior Theory." *Journal of Genetic Counseling* 26, no. 2: 322–30. https://doi.org/10.1007/s10897-016-0023-1.

Biesecker, Barbara B., and Lori H. Erby. 2008. "Adaptation to Living with a Genetic Condition or Risk: A Mini-Review." *Clinical Genetics* 74, no. 5: 401–407. https://doi.org/10.1111/j.1399-0004.2008.01088.x.

Biesecker, Barbara B., Lori H. Erby, Samuel Woolford, Jessica Young Adcock, Julie S. Cohen, Amanda Lamb, . . . Bryce B. Reeve. 2013. "Development and Validation of the Psychological Adaptation Scale (PAS): Use in Six Studies of Adaptation to a Health Condition or Risk." *Patient Education and Counseling* 93, no. 2: 248–54. https://doi.org/10.1016/j.pec.2013.05.006.

Biesecker, Barbara B., and Kathryn F. Peters. 2001. "Process Studies in Genetic Counseling: Peering into the Black Box." *American Journal of Medical Genetics* 106, no. 3: 191–98. https://doi.org/10.1002/ajmg.10004.

Caswell-Jin, J. L., A. D. Zimmer, and W. Stedden. 2019. "Cascade Genetic Testing of Relatives for Hereditary Cancer Risk: Results of an Online Initiative." *Journal of the National Cancer Institute* 111: 95–98. https://doi.org/10.1093/jnci/djy147.

Cheung, E. L., A. D. Olson, T. M. Yu, P. Z. Han, and M. S. Beattie. 2010. "Communication of BRCA Results and Family Testing in 1,103 High-Risk Women." *Cancer Epidemiology, Biomarkers, and Prevention* 19: 2211–19. https://doi.org/10.1158/1055-9965.EPI-10-0325.

Cohen, Julie S., and Barbara B. Biesecker. 2010. "Quality of Life in Rare Genetic Conditions: A Systematic Review of the Literature." *American Journal of Medical Genetics. Part A* 152A, no. 5: 1136–56. https://doi.org/10.1002/ajmg.a.33380.

Dent, K. M., C. Harper, L. Kearney, C. Lieber, and B. Finucane. 2011. "Embracing the Unique Role of Genetic Counselors: Response to the Commentary by Madeo et al." *American Journal of Medical Genetics. Part A* 155A, no. 8: 1791–93. https://doi.org/10.1002/ajmg.a.34111.

Dong, Danielle A. 2005. "Causal Attributions for Autistic Spectrum Disorders: Influences on Perceived Personal Control." Unpublished Master of Science Thesis. Bloomberg School of Public Health of Johns Hopkins University.

Dormandy, E., E. Y. Tsui, and T. M. Marteau. 2007. "Development of a Measure of Informed Choice Suitable for Use in Low Literacy Populations." *Patient Education and Counseling* 66: 278–95. https://doi.org/10.1016/j.pec.2007.01.001.

Duster, Troy. 1990. *Backdoor to Eugenics*. New York: Routledge.

Elrick, Ashley, S. Ashida, J. Ivanovich, S. Lyons, B. Biesecker, M. S. Goodman, and Kimberly A. Kaphingst. 2017. "Psychosocial and Clinical Factors Associated with Family Communication of Cancer Genetic Test Results among Women Diagnosed with Breast Cancer at a Young Age." *Journal of Genetic Counseling* 26, no. 1: 173–81. https://doi.org/10.1007/s10897-016-9995-0.

Evers-Kiebooms, G., and H. van den Berghe. 1979. "Impact of Genetic Counseling: A Review of Published Follow-up Studies." *Clinical Genetics* 15, no. 6: 465–74. http://www.ncbi.nlm.nih.gov/pubmed/380852.

Fanos, Joanna H. 1999a. "The Missing Link in Linkage Analysis: The Well Sibling Revisited." *Genetic Testing* 3, no. 3: 273–78. https://doi.org/10.1089/109065799316581.

Fanos, Joanna H. 1999b. "'My Crooked Vision': The Well Sib Views Ataxia-Telangiectasia." *American Journal of Medical Genetics* 87, no. 5: 420–25. http://www.ncbi.nlm.nih.gov/pubmed/10594881.

Fanos, Joanna H., Susan Gronka, Joanne Wuu, Christine Stanislaw, Peter M. Andersen, and Michael Benatar. 2011. "Impact of Presymptomatic Genetic Testing for Familial Amyotrophic Lateral Sclerosis." *Genetics in Medicine* 13, no. 4: 342–48. https://doi.org/10.1097/GIM.0b013e318204d004.

Fiddler, M. B., B. A. Fine, D. L. Baker, and ABGC Consensus Development Consortium. 1996. "A Case-Based Approach to the Development of Practice-Based Competencies for Accreditation of and Training in Graduate Programs in Genetic Counseling." *Journal of Genetic Counseling* 5, no. 3: 105–12. https://doi.org/10.1007/BF01408655.

Fine, Beth A., Diane L. Baker, and Morris B. Fiddler. 1996. "Practice-Based Competencies for Accreditation of and Training in Graduate Programs in Genetic Counseling." *Journal of Genetic Counseling* 5, no. 3: 113–21. https://doi.org/10.1007/BF01408656.

Fraser, F. C. 1974. "Genetic Counseling." *American Journal of Human Genetics* 27, no. 5: 636–59. http://www.ncbi.nlm.nih.gov/pubmed/4609197.

Grant, P. E., M. Pampaka, K. Payne, A. Clarke and M. McAllster. 2019. Developing a short-form of the Genetic Counselling Outcome Scale: The Genomics Outcome Scale. *European Journal of Medical Genetics* 62, no. 5: 324–334. doi:Epub 2018 Nov 26.

Gray, Stacy W., Sarah E. Gollust, Deanna Alexis Carere, Clara A. Chen, Angel Cronin, Sarah S. Kalia, . . . Robert C. Green. 2017. "Personal Genomic Testing for Cancer Risk: Results from the Impact of Personal Genomics Study." *Journal of Clinical Oncology* 35, no. 6: 636–44. https://doi.org/10.1200/JCO.2016.67.1503.

Green, M. J., A. M. McInerney, B. B. Biesecker, and N. Fost. 2001. "Education about Genetic Testing for Breast Cancer Susceptibility: Patient Preferences for a Computer Program or Genetic Counselor." *American Journal of Medical Genetics* 103, no. 1: 24–31. http://www.ncbi.nlm.nih.gov/pubmed/11562930.

Han Paul K. J., Kendall L. Umstead, Barbara A. Bernhardt, et al. 2017. "A taxonomy of medical uncertainties in clinical genome sequencing." *Genetics in Medicine* 9, no. 8: 918–925. doi:10.1038/gim.2016.212

Katz, A. H. 1963. "Social Adaptation in Chronic Illness: A Study of Hemophilia." *American Journal of Public Health and the Nation's Health* 53 (October): 1666–75. http://www.ncbi.nlm.nih.gov/pubmed/14070736.

Kessler, Seymour. 1979. *Genetic Counseling: Psychological Dimensions.* New York: Academic Press.

Kessler, Seymour. 1997. Psychological Aspects of Genetic Counseling. IX. Teaching and Counseling. *Journal of Genetic Counseling* 6, no. 3: 287–295. doi:10.1023/A:1025676205440

Kumar, Neha, Erin Turbitt, Barbara B. Biesecker, Ilana M. Miller, Breana Cham, Katherine C. Smith, and Rajiv N. Rimal. 2019. Managing the Need to Tell: Triggers and Strategic Disclosure of Thalassemia Major in Singapor. *American Journal of Medical Genetics Part A* 179, no. 5: 762–769.

Lazarus, R. S., and S. Folkman. 1984. *Stress, Appraisal, and Coping. Behaviour Research and Therapy.*

Lippman-Hand, A., and F. C. Fraser. 1979a. "Genetic Counseling—the Postcounseling Period: I. Parents' Perceptions of Uncertainty." *American Journal of Medical Genetics* 4, no. 1: 51–71. https://doi.org/10.1002/ajmg.1320040108.

Lippman-Hand, A., and F. C. Fraser. 1979b. "Genetic Counseling: Parents' Responses to Uncertainty." *Birth Defects Original Article Series* 15, no. 5C: 325–39. http://www.ncbi.nlm.nih.gov/pubmed/526612.

Lippman-Hand, A., and F. C. Fraser. 1979c. "Genetic Counseling: Provision and Reception of Information." *American Journal of Medical Genetics* 3, no. 2: 113–27. https://doi.org/10.1002/ajmg.1320030202.

Lippman-Hand, A., and F. C. Fraser. 1979d. "Genetic Counseling—the Postcounseling Period: II. Making Reproductive Choices." *American Journal of Medical Genetics* 4, no. 1: 73–87. https://doi.org/10.1002/ajmg.1320040109.

Madeo, Anne C., Barbara B. Biesecker, Campbell Brasington, Lori H. Erby, and Kathryn F. Peters. 2011. "The Relationship between the Genetic Counseling Profession and the Disability Community: A Commentary." *American Journal of Medical Genetics. Part A* 155A, no. 8: 1777–85. https://doi.org/10.1002/ajmg.a.34054.

Marteau, T., E. Dormandy, and R. Crockett. 2005. "Informed Choice: Why Measuring Behaviour Is Important." *Archives of Disease in Childhood* 90, no. 5: 546–47.

McAllister, M., and A. Dearing. 2015. "Patient-Reported Outcomes and Patient Empowerment in Clinical Genetics Services." *Clinical Genetics* 88, no. 2: 114–21. https://doi.org/10.1111/cge.12520.

McAllister M., A. M. Wood, G. Dunn, S. Shiloh, C. Todd. 2011. "The Genetic Counseling Outcome Scale: a new patient-reported outcome measure for clinical genetics services." *Clinical Genetics* 79, 413–24.

Meiser, Bettina, and Veronica Quinn. 2018. "Psychological Outcomes and Surgical Decisions after Genetic Testing in Women Newly Diagnosed with Breast Cancer with and without a Family History." *European Journal of Human Genetics* 26: 972–83. https://doi.org/10.1038/s41431-017-0057-3.

Meiser, Bettina, Jennifer Irle, Elizabeth Lobb, Kristin Barlow-Stewart. 2008. "Assessment of the content and process of genetic counseling: a critical review of empirical studies." *Journal of Genetic Counseling* 17, no. 5: 434–451.

Michie, S., T. M. Marteau, and M. Bobrow. 1997. "Genetic Counselling: The Psychological Impact of Meeting Patients' Expectations." *Journal of Medical Genetics* 34, no. 3: 237–241. http://www.ncbi.nlm.nih.gov/pubmed/9132497.

Michie, S., V. McDonald, and T. M. Marteau. 1997. "Genetic Counselling: Information Given, Recall and Satisfaction." *Patient Education and Counseling* 32, no. 1–2: 101–106. http://www.ncbi.nlm.nih.gov/pubmed/9355577.

Myers, B. A., S. B. Friedman, and I. B. Weiner. 1970. "Coping with a Chronic Disability. Psychosocial Observations of Girls with Scoliosis Treated with the Milwaukee Brace." *American Journal of Diseases of Children* 120, no. 3: 175–81. http://www.ncbi.nlm.nih.gov/pubmed/4917851.

Parens, Erik, and Adrienne Asch, eds. 2000. *Prenatal Testing and Disability Rights.* Washington, DC: Georgetown University Press.

Parens, Erik, and Adrienne Asch. 2003. "Disability Rights Critique of Prenatal Genetic Testing: Reflections and Recommendations." *Mental Retardation and Developmental Disabilities Research Reviews* 9, no. 1: 40–47. https://doi.org/10.1002/mrdd.10056.

Peters, Kathryn F., and Stephen A. Petrill. 2011a. "A Comparison of the Background, Needs, and Expectations of Patients Seeking Genetic Counseling Services." *American Journal of Medical Genetics Part A.* 155, no. 4: 697–705. https://doi.org/10.1002/ajmg.a.33979.

Peters, Kathryn F., and Stephen A. Petrill. 2011b. "Comparison of the Background, Needs, and Expectations for Genetic Counseling of Adults with Experience with Down Syndrome, Marfan Syndrome, and Neurofibromatosis." *American Journal of Medical Genetics, Part A* 155, no. 4: 684–696. https://doi.org/10.1002/ajmg.a.33863.

Redlinger-Grosse, Krista, Patricia McCarthy Veach, Bonnie S. LeRoy, and Heather Zierhut. 2017. "Elaboration of the Reciprocal-Engagement Model of Genetic Counseling Practice: A Qualitative Investigation of Goals and Strategies." *Journal of Genetic Counseling* 26, no. 6: 1372–387. https://doi.org/10.1007/s10897-017-0114-7.

Redlinger-Grosse, Krista., Veach, Patricia. McCartthy Veach., Cohen, Stephanie., LeRoy, Bonnie. S., MacFarlane, Ian. M., and Zierhut, Heather. 2016. "Defining our clinical practice: The identification of genetic counseling outcomes utilizing the reciprocal engagement model." *Journal of Genetic Counseling* 25, no. 2: 239–257.

Resta, Robert, Barbara Bowles Biesecker, Robin L. Bennett, Sandra Blum, Susan Estabrooks Hahn, Michelle N. Strecker, and Janet L. Williams. 2006. "A New Definition of Genetic Counseling: National Society of Genetic Counselors' Task Force Report." *Journal of Genetic Counseling* 15, no. 2: 77–83. https://doi.org/10.1007/s10897-005-9014-3.

Shiloh, Shoshana, Orit Avdor, and Richard M. Goodman. 1990. "Satisfaction with Genetic Counseling: Dimensions and Measurement." *American Journal of Medical Genetics* 37, no. 4: 522–29. https://doi.org/10.1002/ajmg.1320370419.

Sorenson, J. R., J. P. Swazey, N. A. Scotch, C. M. Kavanagh, and D. B. Matthews. 1981. "Reproductive Pasts, Reproductive Futures. Genetic Counseling and Its Effectiveness." *Birth Defects Original Article Series* 17, no. 4: 1–192. http://www.ncbi.nlm.nih.gov/pubmed/7326367.

Stern, Alexandra Minna. 2012. *Telling Genes: The Story of Genetic Counseling in America.* Baltimore: Johns Hopkins University Press.

Stevenson, Alan Carruth, and Clare Davison. 1970. *Genetic Counselling.* Philadelphia: Lippincott.

Sulzer, Edward S., Gerald Gurin, Joseph Veroff, and Sheila Feld. 1962. "Americans View Their Mental Health: A Nationwide Interview Survey." *American Journal of Psychology* 75, no. 2: 351. https://doi.org/10.2307/1419652.

Sutton, Erica J., Lauren Rosapep, Karen Ball, Megan Truitt, Barbara Biesecker, Rick Guidotti, and Diane McLean. 2006. "Through the Viewfinder: Positive Exposure a Year Later." *American Journal of Medical Genetics. Part C, Seminars in Medical Genetics* 142C, no. 4: 260–68. https://doi.org/10.1002/ajmg.c.30113.

Tavormina, J. B., Kastner, L. D., Slater, P. M., and Watt, S. L. 1976. "Chronically Ill Children: A Psychologically Deviant Population?" *Journal of Abnormal Child Psychology* 4, no. 99: 99–110.

Taylor, Shelley E. 1983. "Adjustment to Threatening Events: A Theory of Cognitive Adaptation." *American Psychologist* 38, no. 11: 1161–173. https://doi.org/10.1037/0003-066X.38.11.1161.

Turriff, Amy, Howard P. Levy, and Barbara Biesecker. 2015. "Factors Associated with Adaptation to Klinefelter Syndrome: The Experience of Adolescents and Adults." *Patient Education and Counseling* 98, no. 1: 90–95. https://doi.org/10.1016/j.pec.2014.08.012.

Tversky, A., and D. Kahneman. 1974. "Judgment under Uncertainty: Heuristics and Biases." *Science* 185, no. 4157: 1124–131. https://doi.org/10.1126/science.185.4157.1124.

Umstead, Kendall, Sarah S. Kalia, Anne C. Madeo, Lori H. Erby, Thomas O. Blank, Kala Visvanathan, and Debra L. Roter. 2018. "Social comparisons and quality of life following a prostate cancer diagnosis." *Journal of Psychosocial Oncology* 36, no. 3: 350–363. doi:10.1080/07347332.2017.1417950

Veach, Patricia McCarthy, Dianne M. Bartels, and Bonnie S. LeRoy. 2007. "Coming Full Circle: A Reciprocal-Engagement Model of Genetic Counseling Practice." *Journal of Genetic Counseling* 16, no. 6: 713–28. https://doi.org/10.1007/s10897-007-9113-4.

Visotsky, Harold M. 1961. "Coping Behavior under Extreme Stress." *Archives of General Psychiatry* 5, no. 5: 423. https://doi.org/10.1001/archpsyc.1961.01710170001001.

Walker, Ann. 1998. "The Practice of Genetic Counseling." In *A Guide to Genetic Counseling*, edited by Diane L Baker, Jane L Schuette, and Wendy R Uhlman, 1–20. New York: Wiley-Liss.

Weisman, A. D., and H. J. Sobel. 1979. "Coping with Cancer through Self-Instruction: A Hypothesis." *Journal of Human Stress* 5, no. 1: 3–8. https://doi.org/10.1080/0097840X.1979.9934997.

Wertz, D. C., and J. C. Fletcher. 1988. "Ethics and Medical Genetics in the United States: A National Survey." *American Journal of Medical Genetics* 29, no. 4: 815–27. https://doi.org/10.1002/ajmg.1320290411.

Wertz, D. C., and R. Gregg. 2000. "Genetics Services in a Social, Ethical and Policy Context: A Collaboration Between Consumers and Providers." *Journal of Medical Ethics* 26: 261–265.

Wortman, Camille B., and Roxane C. Silver. 1989. "The Myths of Coping with Loss." *Journal of Consulting and Clinical Psychology* 57, no. 3: 349–57. https://doi.org/10.1037/0022-006X.57.3.349.

Zierhut, Heather A., K. M. Shannon, Debra. L. Cragun, Stephanie. A. Cohen. 2016. Elucidating Genetic Counseling Outcomes from the Perspective of Genetic Counselors. *Journal of Genetic Counseling* 25, no. 5: 993–1001. doi:10.1007/s10897-015-9930-9

CHAPTER 4

Characteristics of Genetic Counseling Clients

The most formidable but rewarding part of genetic counseling happens when you sit down with clients and begin the process of helping them integrate genetic information into their lives as they try to invest it with psychological and emotional meaning. We aim to make this experience less intimidating by examining some of the sociological, demographic, and biological factors that help shape each client into a unique human being.

In this chapter, we explore how the ways that the genetic counselor, consciously or subconsciously, perceives the fundamental biological, social, and cultural characteristics traits of counselees can have a significant effect on the dynamics of the genetic counseling session and ultimately on the quality of services that are delivered.

Our intent is not so much to exhaustively review each of these characteristics but instead to heighten your sensitivity to them so that you can be a more self-aware genetic counselor. Studies have shown that counselors who are aware of their sensitivity to their clients' characteristics are able to more effectively care for their clients (McCalman et al. 2017). These traits often raise a dynamic of transference and countertransference between genetic counselor and client. You should familiarize yourself with the concepts of transference and countertransference by reviewing Chapter 5 on advanced counseling skills.

We cannot overemphasize the importance of clinical supervision across your genetic counseling career, from novice to highly experienced genetic counselors. An effective supervisor can help you gain a professional and more objective perspective on your patient interactions by post-session analysis and dissection. This is a critical aspect of your professional growth.

It is a never-ending process even for the most experienced and enlightened genetic counselor, Audio-recording of your sessions can be a powerful way to increase your self-awareness of your counseling techniques (see Chapter 5 for more discussion about audio-recording).

WHAT'S IN A NAME?

What is the proper term for people who seek genetic counseling? We can probably agree that the term *counselee*, while technically accurate, is somewhat awkward and stilted, and is not used very often in common practice outside of the context of research studies. More often, the terms *patient* and *client* are used. Some genetic counselors have fairly strong feelings and preferences for one term over the other, with perhaps a stronger emotional attachment to *client* rather than *patient*. Let's look at the words more closely.

Patient is a time-honored term for people receiving medical care; its use, according to the Oxford English Dictionary, goes back to at least Chaucer's time. Many genetic counselors work in a clinical setting, where colleagues use the term frequently, and so its use is natural in this setting. Certainly, many people who seek genetic counseling have serious diseases and referring to them as *patients* is accurate. And many other health professionals—physicians, nurse practitioners, physician assistants, etc.—use the term *patient* even though the vast majority of the people they see are healthy and are typically seen for routine physicals, blood tests, or health screening.

Client, on the other hand, suggests that genetic counseling is something more than a standard medical encounter. Many counselees are not seeking disease treatment. They may be pregnant or investigating their family history of cancer or experiencing infertility or seeking to learn about recurrence risks or seeking a diagnosis for their child, but many are not in a disease state (at least, not yet). *Client* also helps distinguish genetic counseling from medical genetics, where a primary goal is to diagnose and perhaps treat a disease.

Sometimes it becomes difficult to decide when to call someone a *patient* and when to call someone a *client*. For example, what about a woman who undergoes repeat breast biopsies to determine if a lesion is malignant or benign? Or a man who has fifteen colon polyps detected on a screening colonoscopy? Or a presymptomatic thirty-five-year-old with a 45 repeat CAG expansion in the *HTT* gene who is nearly certain to develop symptoms of Huntington disease in the next five to ten years? A person's status may change from client to patient over time. Consider the case of an asymptomatic man who has a pathogenic variant in the *MLH1* gene that is diagnostic for Lynch syndrome, at which point he would be a client, but then develops colon cancer, at which point he would become a patient.

Some genetic counselors work primarily with people who are affected by a disease, in which case the word *patient* is likely to be used frequently. Some genetic counselors work with people who are not particularly likely to have a genetic disease, such as in a prenatal setting, in which case *client* may be more commonly used. But many genetic counselors work with a roughly equal mix of healthy and affected clients, such as in a hereditary cancer clinic, and switching back and forth between *client* and *patient* becomes difficult.

On the other hand, *client* also carries economic connotations. Bankers, advertising agencies, talent agents, corporate lawyers, and investment firms refer to those who use their services as *clients*. This can subtly suggest that genetic counselors view people as a source of income and could rob the encounter of its rich psychological and human component. This is not a trivial matter in light of the trend at many medical institutions to push for a Customer Service Model of patient care. People seeking medical care, in our view, should be treated with compassion, skill, and respect; in contrast, customers are just people we view as a source of income.

At the end of the day, it probably does not matter that much if you use *patient* or *client*, or, like many genetic counselors, you use both interchangeably in your daily practice. But broadly speaking, we tend to reserve *clients* for healthy people undergoing genetic counseling and *patients* for affected individuals undergoing genetic counseling. We, however, reject the terms *customer* and *consumer* (Krugman 2011).

CLIENT CHARACTERISTICS

Although it may seem self-evident that patients' age, gender, culture, and other demographic and personal factors influence the genetic counseling process and encounter, there is a surprising dearth of research that addresses this within the context of genetic counseling specifically. Most of the research explores the impact of these factors on the outcome of genetic counseling. There are few studies of how the genetic counselor's or the patient's perception of those factors influences the dynamics of the genetic counseling session. The lack of evidence makes it difficult to follow evidence-based guidelines that address this important relational issue.

Although this chapter divides patients into categories for simplicity of highlighting characteristics that may affect genetic counseling, we strongly encourage you to be very wary of thinking about patients in terms of categories. Typological thinking can be very difficult to avoid, especially when it comes to gender, race, and socioeconomic status. This is easier said than done. Think of the whole set of preconceptions evoked by the mythical stereotypes "upper-class white male bond fund trader" versus "lower-class black female single mother of five on government assistance." We and our patients are socialized to think of each other as belonging to semi-rigid categories that behave in a certain way—men, religious fundamentalists, drug abusers, lesbians, poor people, college educated, high school dropout, etc. Such categories often tell us more about who is doing the pigeonholing and what issues are driving the categorization process.

How we define ourselves—and others—is strongly dependent on context. If you are speaking to a fellow genetic counselor, you might describe yourself as a cancer genetic counselor or a prenatal counselor. To a physician, you would say that you are a genetic counselor. In a political discussion, you might say that you are a liberal, or a libertarian, or a conservative. If you are visiting another city, you might describe yourself by the name of your city of residence. If you are spending time in another country, you would probably identify yourself as a citizen of your home country. From an ethnic standpoint, you would define yourself by the ethnicity of your forebears. Socially you might identify by your gender or age group. Each of these categories captures some aspect of you, but none captures all of you. In turn, the perception of you by others is refracted through the prism of their personal experiences with genetic counselors, religious faith, political leanings, geographic residence, socioeconomic status, etc.

Within any of these identities there is so much variability that the categories themselves can become meaningless. To further complicate the picture, the various categories interact and influence one another. A patient can be a thirty-five-year-old ultra-orthodox Jewish woman who was born in Russia and migrated to the United States when she was twenty-five, who speaks minimal English, whose husband is a businessman, who has severe pain from adult-onset Gaucher disease, and who is pregnant with her eighth child. All of these factors interact in complicated ways during the genetic counseling encounter, and it is quite difficult to separate them. Indeed, they are not separate entities, and to treat them as such is a basic misunderstanding and misreading of human behavior and psychology.

It is the job of the genetic counselor, not of the patient, to avoid stereotyping, or, more precisely, for the genetic counselor to identify when the counseling is influenced by the counselor's preconceptions. The ability to recognize the effects of preconceived notions on the genetic counseling encounter requires a combination of experience, self-awareness, continuing education, and supervision. The interplay of transference and countertransference that results from basic differences between counselor and counselee is an unavoidable occurrence of any interaction between two human beings. Becoming aware of this dynamic, and not letting it negatively influence the delivery of genetic counseling, is a critical skill to develop and requires constant work throughout one's professional career (see Chapter 5). Even more complex are the implicit biases we all have that may influence our relationships with clients in ways we are less cognizant of (Schaa et al. 2015).

CROSS-CULTURAL GENETIC COUNSELING

The terms *race, ethnicity,* and *culture* are often used as if they have clear meaning and distinction. The terms are frequently used in the media, government reports, and academic publications. Yet all three defy precise definition and are not uncommonly used almost interchangeably. Indeed, it is often argued that race has no biological basis (Templeton 2013) and is entirely a social construct whose parameters tell us more about the definers than the defined (Graves 2002). One way to think about these terms is to view race as certain biological characteristics that can be loosely associated with skin color; ethnicity as group identification that is somewhat based on race; and culture as the behaviors, beliefs, and norms that characterize an ethnic group. But, quite frankly, the world does not fit into neat little packages, and losing sight of this will only result in substandard genetic counseling, from both a biomedical, a psychological, and a social perspective.

Interactions among race, ethnicity, and culture are further complicated by cultural history and socioeconomic status (SES) (Williams et al. 2010). Past experiences with health care and other authorities can affect interactions with genetic counselors. For example, ethnicity and SES may influence the decision to continue a pregnancy in which a sex chromosome abnormality was diagnosed (Jeon et al. 2012). Non-Whites who were provided telephone counseling about BRCA testing were less likely to undergo testing than Whites (Butrick et al. 2015). African American women tend to have higher levels of mistrust of the medical system in general (Sheppard et al. 2013) and have poorer survival from breast cancer than White women even though they face a lower lifetime risk of developing the disease (Hsu et al. 2017). This is the result of a complicated blend of biology, medicine, and socioeconomic factors that are extraordinarily difficult to separate— and maybe they should not be separated, as it may result in treating them as discrete entities and emphasizing one over the others (Daly and Olopade 2015). Low SES and race are associated with likelihood of referral, adherence to medical recommendations, stage at presentation of disease, comorbidities, prognosis, and local availability of health care, particularly when it comes to high-tech medical interventions (Cragun et al. 2015).

In a study of hypertrophic cardiomyopathy from Australia, the highest rates of nonadherence with medication usage were associated with younger age, minority ethnicity, anxiety, and poor mental quality of life (Ingles et al. 2015). The authors concluded that "Of all the patients attending a specialized cardiac genetic clinic, there is an overrepresentation of patients from very advantaged and major metropolitan areas and [this] suggests that those most in need of a multidisciplinary approach to care are not accessing it" (Ingles et al. 2015, p. 743).

Most genetic counselors in the United States, Canada, the United Kingdom, Australia, and New Zealand are females from the dominant Northern and Western European White culture. Particularly in the United States, this is a disproportionately large segment compared to the ethnic structure of the population (National Society of Genetic Counselors 2018). But the following discussion applies to all genetic counselors, regardless of their ethnocultural heritage. For the most part, since they have lived a life primarily among their own culture and socioeconomic group, the cultural training of genetic counselors should focus on training them to be aware of their beliefs and biases.

There is also a common but nonverbalized tendency to view other cultures as if they belong in a *National Geographic* television special where, paradoxically, others can be simultaneously perceived as exotically interesting and distastefully different. Being judgmental is a common and natural behavior. Genetic counselors are, at the end of the day, people and should not be blamed for this widely shared human trait. However, counselors must be aware of when their personal views are negatively influencing genetic counseling encounters.

Knowledge of Other Cultures

Unless a genetic counselor works exclusively and exhaustively with one small segment of the population, it is unrealistic to expect him or her to have an encyclopedic knowledge of the sociocultural characteristics, beliefs, attitudes, etc. of all of their patients. Most clinics serve too diverse a patient population for genetic counselors to develop such knowledge. In many cases, "book knowledge" of sociocultural issues does not directly translate into effective clinical encounters. Cultural clashes, where the counselor may unintentionally and inadvertently violate a social norm of a client or where a client or the counselor may misinterpret words and behaviors differently, are inevitable. The aim is to minimize their occurrence and to work through them in ways that result in clients receiving the best possible care.

A genetic counseling session from one of our own practices (Resta) illuminates the ways that cultural differences can create an awkward situation. Once, when working in a prenatal diagnosis clinic, he met with a Native American woman and her husband who was also Native American but with a different tribal affiliation than his wife. The session began typically enough: We discussed why they came to the clinic and what they wanted to get out of the session. The woman did all of the speaking up to this point; her husband remained quiet. As Resta began to ask questions about family history, the husband rose to his full and impressive height, angrily announced, "This is bullshit!" and marched out of the office and right out of the clinic. At this point, the counselor was in internal panic mode, totally at a loss about what he had just done to evoke such a reaction and what he should do next. Prior to this, he had experience with several patients storming out of his office, but he could usually identify the behavior as an understandable reaction to some very intense and unanticipated medical news, or, in a few cases, as an attempt at emotional manipulation of the partner. But in this particular situation, he grasped for an explanation.

Fortunately, the wife stayed in the room. He looked at her half-helplessly and asked her what was going on and what she thought may have sparked the outburst. She replied, with a half-smile, "Oh, he can just be a real jerk sometimes. Don't pay any attention to him." The counselor gave her a slight nod that silently thanked her for allowing him not to feel too terrible and to permit him to resume a normal breathing pattern. She explained that in his tribe, a now small and poverty-stricken people, members never speak about their ancestors to outsiders, and most especially not to the dominant culture of relatively affluent white men. Out of respect for her husband, she did not want to supply details about gender, specific relationships, ages, and causes of death about his relatives. She did feel comfortable, though, answering broad questions about his family history with regards to developmental delays, physical disabilities, and other items of interest to a genetic counselor because she could see the relevance of the information to her appointment.

In the end, this genetic counseling session more or less worked out for both the patient and the counselor because of the open-mindedness and support of the wife. But there is no way the counselor could have been prepared for this; he had not knowingly encountered another member of this tribe previously or since that time. The clinic's usual practice was to send patients an appointment letter that explained what would happen during genetic counseling, and this could have helped address this situation up front as it would have given the husband the opportunity to explain his beliefs at the outset. Unfortunately, in this case, the appointment had been set up urgently for the next morning and so a letter would not reach the client prior to the appointment.

On the other hand, we have also had a few patients from our own white European background refuse to provide their family history because they were convinced that the information would go into "the government's database" and would be used against them. Interestingly, most were male, and all used the same term to describe this alleged nefarious cabal. Resta internally dismissed these men as paranoid oddballs, whereas his experience with the Native American male in the example above made him feel he was disrespectful because he had violated a deep cultural taboo. Considering these cases forced him to realize that he also viewed his own culture through a biased lens.

In one study, genetic counselors who displayed an implicit pro-White bias as measured by the Race Implicit Association Test tended to use less emotionally responsive communication and lower levels of positive affect when counseling minorities (Schaa et al. 2015). We encourage all genetic counselors to take this online test at https://implicit.harvard.edu/implicit/ . You will likely learn that it is indeed very difficult to recognize and overcome our unconscious biases.

Nonetheless, if a genetic counselor's client population includes more than a sprinkling of patients from the nondominant culture, it is helpful to be alert to the broad outlines of certain cultural and religious issues. Counselors should be aware of the range of behaviors and beliefs of these clients out of respect for their client's sense of identity and personal values and to allow the business of genetic counseling to take place in a manner that the client finds supportive and helpful, despite cultural and socioeconomic differences between counselor and counselee. Of course, genetic counselors should not stereotypically expect their clients from these cultures to behave in these ways, but they should be fully prepared for such behaviors and beliefs to be part of the genetic counseling encounter (Weil 2000).

Some examples that illustrate this include:

- Ultra-Orthodox Jews who say they are *shomer negiah*, "observant of touch," adhering to the teaching that forbids shaking of hands between men and women (Mittman et al. 2007). Let the ultra-Orthodox client initiate a handshake if he or she sees fit; don't create an awkward moment by being the first to extend your hand in greeting.
- The reluctance of some Amish clients to pose for photos, especially portraits, as it conflicts with their commitment to humility and violates the biblical ban on graven images (http://www.discoverlancaster.com/towns-and-heritage/amish-country/amish-and-photographs.asp).

Don't unthinkingly take out a camera to photograph an Amish child in a dysmorphology clinic without first explaining to the parent what you want to do and seek their approval.
- Some groups prefer not to sign consent forms as they believe their oral assent to be sufficient and see a request for a signature as disregarding the trustworthiness of their word (Lakes et al. 2012). Work with your institution to develop policies that allow flexibility for different ways of providing informed consent to meet the needs of different clients.
- The common preference of Muslim women to be examined by a female provider (Vu et al. 2016). Muslim women should be asked if they have a preference for provider gender when an appointment is set up.
- The importance of family and elders in making important decisions among people from many parts of East Asia (Hobbs et al. 2015). Encourage parents, aunts, grandparents, or other important elders to attend the genetic counseling session and let them express their views or encourage your patients to go home and discuss the relevant genetic counseling issues with other family members as they see fit.

There are plenty of resources on the internet and in libraries that offer both brief and in-depth information on the sociocultural characteristics, demographics, and economic status of the many cultures that coexist in many countries with both longstanding and recent histories of migrant populations, forced or otherwise. If you work with more than the usual share of patients from these communities, it would be in your best interests to avail yourself of these resources.

Language

Ideally, genetic counselors should be able to speak the language of their clients to ensure accurate transmission of genetic information and to engage the client in psychologically meaningful relationship, but the vast majority of genetic counselors are fluent only in English. Thus, professional interpreters play a critical role. At least one study has shown that, for better or worse, the interpreter can influence Latinas' decisions about undergoing amniocentesis (Preloran et al. 2005). Most patients are usually better served by a professional interpreter than an untrained interpreter (Flores et al. 2012; Hunt and deVoogd 2007; Karliner et al. 2007; Nápoles et al. 2015; Raymond 2014). Most medical centers require use of a professional interpreter when counseling someone who is not comfortable communicating in English, and in the United States, Title VI of the Civil Rights Act of 1964 makes this a legal requirement for institutions receiving federal funds (Office for Civil

Rights Policy Guidance n.d.). This policy does not always sit well with some families, who may prefer to use a close relative or friend as a translator. The patient may have legitimate reasons for such a request—translators may be from their social community and thus the patients may feel that their confidentiality is being compromised despite assurances of the professional obligations of the interpreter, female patients may feel less comfortable discussing sexual and pregnancy issues with a male interpreter, or the patient may place greater trust in the friend or relative than a stranger. This can put the genetic counselor in the awkward position of having to adhere to institutional policy at the risk of alienating patients, although the Office for Civil Rights Policy Guidance is clear that patients do not have to be forced to use a professional interpreter. A potential solution in some situations is to simultaneously utilize both the close relative and the professional in interpretation roles. That is, let the relative serve as the primary translator but use the professional interpreter for complex medical discussions. This allows the genetic counselor to monitor the overall accuracy of the translation while relieving the relative of the burden of translating sophisticated medical terminology. Many genetic counselors have had the experience of having had a complex medical discussion transformed by a nonprofessional interpreter into a brief sentence in the native language of the patient. This would be a good time to check in with the professional interpreter.

Another language difference situation arises when both partners are fluent in English and medically sophisticated and clearly do not need a professional interpreter. Many genetic counselors have had the experience of such a couple, at various points during the session, carry on an extended discussion with each other in their native tongue. For whatever reasons, the couple has excluded the counselor from their discussion. Sometimes they are simply checking in with each other to make sure that they are both understanding what the counselor was saying to them. But other times rich psychological and social issues and subtle relationship interactions are made invisible to the counselor, perhaps at the preference of the clients. In such situations, we have found it is usually best to respect the couple's preferences, but if the discussion continues in their native language then it is best to ask the couple what they are discussing because you want to see if there is something else that you can do to facilitate communication and discussion.

Gender

Far more women than men undergo genetic counseling and testing, even for conditions such as Lynch syndrome that affect both genders equally

(Sharaf et al. 2013). To a large extent, this reflects that men do not get pregnant and a goodly portion of genetic counseling is grounded in reproductive issues. In addition, men are much less likely to seek medical care than women (Pinkhasov et al. 2010). But this disparity is also a function of recordkeeping in genetic counseling clinics. Although many men attend genetic counseling sessions with their female partners, they are not "counted" in clinic statistics even though they may be equally active participants in the process and outcome of genetic counseling.

In subtle and unconscious ways, taken together these factors can result in the counselor focusing on the woman rather than the couple, or downplaying the role of the partner during the genetic counseling session. Nonetheless, it is typically the pregnant female patient who is referred by the obstetric care provider, and the health insurer (in countries without universal health care) pays for a visit in the woman's name, not the man's name, even if the insurance policy holder is the male. Moreover, the roles of men in the process and the outcomes of genetic counseling are less well studied, or, when they are studied, tend to be considered within the context of a couple rather than as a separate participant in genetic counseling.

Not uncommonly, men as the primary clients attend cancer genetic counseling at the request of family members (Lobb et al. 2009; Strømsvik et al. 2009) rather than at their own initiative (Daly 2009). Men found to carry BRCA mutations display many of the same emotional concerns that female carriers display—fears about their own cancer risks and the risks that their offspring face (Strømsvik, Råheim, and Gjengedal 2011); they have specific emotional and educational needs that should be addressed (Graves et al. 2011; Shiloh et al. 2013); and they may have fewer emotional support networks than women (Strømsvik et al. 2010). A study of Finnish men undergoing BRCA-related genetic counseling found that while most men were satisfied with the technical genetic counseling content, about half of the men felt that the counselor did not adequately address the role of social support. Men may also be less likely to be the primary communicators of genetic information within families (Batte et al. 2015), but this is not a universal finding (Finlay et al. 2008).

Men may also be less likely to have genetic test results communicated to them within families (Montgomery et al. 2013) and less likely to undergo genetic testing, and the paternal lineage may be perceived to be less at risk for hereditary breast/ovarian cancer (Evans et al. 2009; Finlay et al. 2008). The traditional roles of fathers in different cultures and attitudes toward discussions between father and son of sex-related health issues also can influence communication about hereditary risks (Hicks, Litwin, and Maliski 2014).

The client's gender can also evoke subtle transference and countertransference issues between client and counselor. In particular, the genetic counselor's personal experience with relationships—partner, parent, lover, spouse, boyfriend, girlfriend, sibling—can influence how the client or the client's partner is perceived. This may be particularly true if the counselor has had negative or traumatic experiences in relationships. This may very well occur on a subconscious level and require professional supervision to appreciate how past personal experience influences the dynamics and process of the genetic counseling encounter. This is yet one more aspect of genetic counseling that is ripe for research.

A few countries are inching toward wider acceptance of individuals who do not fit feel they fit neatly into dichotomous gender categories of male or female. This will likely result in genetic counselors working with patients whose gender identity is fluid. Do such individuals have unique needs and issues in the context of genetic counseling? In one study, less than 20% of genetic counselors reported training in lesbian/gay/bisexual/questioning/transgender (LGBQT+) issues (Glessner et al. 2012). Openness and sensitivity are important for people of all gender identities, and some genetic counselors may benefit from additional sensitivity training in gender identity. One area where this may be particularly salient is genetic counseling of clients of nontraditional gender identification who are at increased hereditary risk of developing uterine, ovarian, breast, or prostate cancer. Individuals of one phenotype who are partially or completely transitioning to another gender identity can have understandably complex questions about appropriate surgeries—prostatectomy, breast reduction, hormone treatment, oophorectomy, hysterectomy—and it can get quite complex to keep straight which organs clients were born with, which body parts they wish to remove, which organs they wish to modify, and which organs they wish to add.

Furthermore, for some individuals, which gender they identify with can determine whether they qualify for coverage of genetic testing. Some insurers have different coverage criteria for males than for females. An individual may be chromosomally female but identify as male and may have some personal difficulty indicating that they are female on the test request form, even though this might allow them to meet criteria for coverage of genetic counseling. And for some patients of fluid gender, their desired body image may change over time. In addition, given the long history of discrimination against non-heterosexuals and disparities in health care experienced by non-traditionally gendered individuals (Makadon 2011), genetic counselors need to create a safe and nonjudgmental environment for LGBQT+ individuals such that they feel comfortable discussing their sexuality and their appropriate genetic counseling needs can be met (VandenLangenberg et al. 2012).

Health Status

The medical status of patients can influence their ability to cognitively and emotionally process the information and psychological issues raised during genetic counseling sessions. Patients' health status can result in emotions and behaviors that initially appear to be unrelated to the immediate genetic counseling issues at hand. For example, in the context of genetic counseling with women who are in the early stages of pregnancy, nausea and tiredness may impair patients' ability to process and remember information and reduce discussion of psychological and social issues. Genetic counselors must be flexible in their counseling plan, taking into account that the symptoms of pregnancy may necessitate breaks in the counseling or a shorter session with follow-up of special issues. Patients should be encouraged to bring along a support person who can serve as a note taker and "second set of ears" to help the patient process the information and emotional issues later on in the comfort of their own homes.

Similarly, patients undergoing chemotherapy may experience impaired memory, cognitive deficits, and poor executive function, so-called chemo brain (Moore 2014). These effects may persist for some time after the end of chemotherapy. Providing genetic counseling to such patients can be quite challenging. The patient may not hear what the counselor says or may not process what is explained; the patient may quickly forget what has been said. Moreover, as with pregnant women, chemotherapy may induce nausea to the point where the patient just wants to bolt from the office; in fact, it might be appropriate to do just that. In such situations, the standard fare of a genetic counseling session may not be an immediate priority for patients. There are very few situations where genetic counseling about hereditary cancer issues cannot wait for a later date.

In some instances, the condition affecting the patient can itself impair cognition, memory, executive function, or perception. This point is particularly germane to patients affected by neurogenetic and psychiatric conditions (Gleichgerrcht et al. 2010). For example, even patients with prodromal Huntington disease experience a wide range of psychiatric and cognitive problems (Epping et al. 2016; Paulsen, Smith, and Long 2013). Many neurological disorders are associated with poor social cognitive function—the ability to process social information and to respond properly to the emotions of others (Henry et al. 2016). Logorrhea—excessively detailed extreme wordiness often about irrelevant matters—can be a side effect of some psychiatric drugs such as the commonly prescribed central nervous system stimulant methylphenidate (commonly marketed as Ritalin in the United States). This can make for a long and complicated session as it is difficult to get such patients focused on the relevant genetic counseling issues. Individuals diagnosed with schizophrenia and bipolar disorder not uncommonly make poor decisions (Cáceda, Nemeroff, and Harvey 2014). Consultation with a psychiatrist may provide insight in how to help these patients make decisions based on genetic information and test results.

Chronic pain is a debilitating problem for patients with genetic disorders such as epidermolysis bullosa, sickle cell anemia, hemophilia, Gaucher disease and other lysosomal storage diseases, Ehlers-Danlos syndrome, and hereditary pancreatitis, to name just a few. People with chronic pain are more likely to experience depression, anxiety, hostility, and poor general emotional functioning (Burke, Mathias, and Denson 2015). In addition, the medications used to manage chronic pain such as opioids can negatively influence verbal fluency, risk-taking behavior, and working verbal memory (Baldacchino et al. 2012). Recognition of these effects can help the genetic counselor understand otherwise puzzling aspects of patients' behaviors, responses, and choices during genetic counseling sessions. The input of pain management specialists can be particularly helpful.

Age

Genetic counselors work with patients across the lifespan, from young children at risk for disorders like familial adenomatous polyposis to octogenarians with breast cancer who are considering genetic testing to help establish the hereditary cancer risks for their children and grandchildren. This wide age range requires an appreciation that certain counseling techniques that are appropriate and effective for patients of one age group might not necessarily be effective in another age group. Genetic counselors should remain open to trying new and varied methods in order to provide genetic counseling for patients of all age groups.

For example, counseling adolescents typically requires a different approach then counseling adults, generally one with more flexibility (Austin 2010; Duncan and Young 2013; Sullivan and McConkie-Rosell 2010; Tercyak 2010). Unfortunately, there is very little research about the most effective way to provide genetic counseling to adolescents. Adolescents typically are developing a sense of personal identity, trying to establish a body image that can fluctuate unpredictably between self-love and self-loathing, and experimenting with different personalities. They may be wary of adults and authority figures. When working with adolescents, genetic counselors need to establish a nonjudgmental relationship and make it clear that any emotions and information that the patient shares are acceptable, safe, and confidential. They should be treated with the same respect and dignity as adults. In their own minds, many adolescents think of themselves as adults, and treating them as such can go a long way to creating a mutually trusting counseling relationship. It is also important to clarify with adolescent client to what extent they desire parental involvement. For all their rebelliousness and resentment of their parents that teens may express verbally, many adolescents want their parents to be part of the genetic counseling process (Syzbowska et al. 2007).

In cancer genetics clinics, it is not uncommon to work with older patients who are undergoing genetic testing to help establish the hereditary cancer risks for their families. Typically, such patients find their way into the office after their adult child met with a genetic counselor to assess his or her hereditary cancer risks. They may have been told that in order to accurately assess the genetic risks in the family, the elderly parent with a personal history of cancer would be the necessary starting point for genetic testing. Working with septuagenarians and older can present a unique set of issues. Older clients may not fully appreciate why they should undergo genetic testing. A common refrain is "Well, why don't you just test my daughter? I've already had cancer. What good is it going to do me to be tested?"

Older clients may have multiple health issues unrelated to their genetic condition—hypertension, cardiac disease, diabetes, physical frailty—that can make it difficult for them to sit for an hour-long genetic counseling session, never mind absorb and process complex genetic information. Memory loss and impairment can make it difficult to remember events from long ago; some family members may have died a half-century or more ago. Genetics may not have been part of their educational curriculum, and terms like *mutation, gene,* and *chromosome* may have only the slimmest of meaning to them. In some situations, such as when an older adult has signs of dementia, the counselor may even question the ability of the patient to provide informed consent.

On the other hand, septuagenarians and older may be quite sharp and interested in learning as much as possible about the genetics of their condition. Almost universally, they have a strong desire to help their children and grandchildren. It is usually helpful to have a family member accompany the clients. Parents and offspring understand each other better than anybody else, and having both present can provide a supportive environment where adult children can interact with their parents and help them understand the reasons for testing the parent.

Genetic counselors need to be aware that age differences between counselor and counselee can evoke countertransference issues and feelings of inadequacy and insecurity on the part of the counselor and the client. This is analogous to patients and genetic counselors who believe that they are better served by, or provide better service to, people from their own ethnic and cultural background. Feelings of inadequacy may arise when very young counselors might feel intimidated by, or unable to connect with, patients who are as old as their parents and grandparents, or older counselors may be unconsciously paternalistic with clients who are young enough to be their children or their grandchildren. Both younger and older genetic counselors may feel that they are not being taken seriously by their patients who are considerably different in age from them.

Countertransference issues could arise from counselors' relationships with their own children, parents, and grandchildren that are unconsciously injected into the genetic counseling dynamic. This hypothetical case helps to illustrate this:

> A nineteen-year-old single nulliparous woman has a strong family history of breast cancer, including her mother, two maternal aunts, three maternal cousins, and her maternal grandmother. Her mother died of metastatic breast cancer at age thirty, when the patient was eight years old. The nineteen-year-old undergoes genetic testing and is found to carry a pathogenic *BRCA1* mutation. When the counselor notifies the patient of her results, she emphatically states that she wants a bilateral mastectomy right away and requests a referral to a breast surgeon. The counselor makes her best attempts to discuss the patient's anxiety and upset at the test results and offers a referral to a psychotherapist or other counseling professional, but the patient still insists on the surgery.

The counselor's countertransference reaction to the patient's situation will be filtered through, among other things, the counselor's personal and familial experience as a teenager. A genetic counselor who is in her or his twenties might subconsciously process this as "Well, I was a mature person at nineteen and made some very difficult adult decisions. Nineteen-year-olds are more mature than many people think, and thus I believe my patient is making a thoughtful and appropriate decision."

Alternatively, the counselor might think, "Jeez, did I make some bad decisions as a teenager! I still acutely regret some of them. This patient's decision is the same kind of bad. I'd better try to talk her out of having a mastectomy."

On the other hand, genetic counselors in their fifties might react differently than younger counselors. One possible subconscious processing might be "My kids were difficult teens and they made more than a few bad decisions. I am embarrassed to admit to myself that my daughter dropped out of high school, and my son dabbled in some bad drugs. This kid thinks she is an adult, but she is just one more dumb teen making one more dumb decision. I almost want to slap her upside her head to knock some sense into her. This is major irreversible surgery. She will lose sensation to her nipples. She will not be able to breastfeed any babies she might have. How can I talk her out of a mastectomy?"

Alternatively, an older counselor might process the situation through this filter: "Well, my kids made some decisions as teens that I thought were pretty bad, but they turned out to be not so bad and even sometimes good decisions. I should help her act on her mastectomy decision."

Many people would judge mastectomy in a nineteen-year-old to be an extreme and possibly inappropriate response to her fears. Some adolescents have difficulty with abstract reasoning and understanding long-term consequences (Callard, Williams, and Skirton 2012). Some nineteen-year-olds are closer to being adults and some are still closer to being teens.

In fact, there probably is no right or wrong decision for this patient, as long as she is fully cognizant of the many implications of undergoing a mastectomy at such a young age. The genetic counselor here needs to be alert to the countertransference process and to help make the patient aware of those implications and understand what meaning they may have for her. Just as importantly, the counselor should explore the patient's lived experience of her mother dying from breast cancer when the patient was at such a developmentally vulnerable age, as well as the background of having so many relatives live—or not—through the breast cancer experience. This is the key work of genetic counseling: to help the client make as informed a decision as she is capable of making at the time.

The ability to attend to a patient's emotional and informational needs, supplemented with professional supervision (see Chapter 5) as appropriate, should overcome any concerns about the potential for inadequacy or countertransference issues leading to a poor genetic counseling session.

Family Dynamics

Everyone has a preconceived notion of what constitutes a family. For many people of Northern and Western European ancestry, the term *family* conjures up an image of mother, father, and the children they conceived together by natural means. Think of what a standard stylized pedigree looks like—a circle and square connected by a horizontal line that is itself attached to another line with more circles and squares hanging neatly off it. It's a nice and pleasing symmetric arrangement of geometric shapes. But if you have drawn even a few pedigrees in the clinic, you quickly realize that many pedigrees resemble complicated abstract paintings of lines with an array of angles, a few hooks thrown in for good measure, and circles and squares sprouting in the darnedest places. This complexity is particularly common when working with highly inbred families or if you are working with couples and clients using assisted reproduction techniques to conceive, where the gestational, genetic, and social parents may be different individuals.

Families are messy in their structure and in their interactions. And they are fluid. Relationships fall apart and reform. Siblings, spouses, and parents are close at some points in their lives and estranged at others. Somehow the genetic counselor must establish how a family is functioning at the moment that they are in the genetics clinic. Who is the patient in the family? How do they make decisions? How does information flow in the family? Who will I stay in touch with long term if the patient is expected to die in the near future?

Genetic counselors work with families from two perspectives. First, from a genetics standpoint, families are a vehicle for the transmission and sharing of genes and hereditary risk. This is why, when taking a pedigree, the counselor seeks to elicit as much relevant biomedical information as possible—health status, age of onset of disease, surgical history, distinguishing between full and half-siblings, cousins, etc. Second, the family is also critical from a psychological and social perspective. The counselor's personal family experiences and concept of what constitutes an ideal family affect both how the counselor provides genetic information and how the patient interprets it, both during the session and future decisions based on that counseling. Further, the information that the counselor imparts is typically about family members because, of course, the information has important medical implications for relatives. How that information is shared plays out against the backdrop of the family's functional and dysfunctional dynamics.

Eliciting a family history and transforming it into a pedigree can reveal much medical information but also provide insights for the counselor and the client into family relationships and stresses. This dual function of a pedigree is what makes it so critical to genetic counseling. We cannot overemphasize the importance of being able to simultaneously elicit both biomedical and psychological and social information when piecing together a family history. Although we fully appreciate the time savings and efficiency achieved by having clients report family histories using an online or paper form prior to their appointments, much richness is lost in the process.

In working with families, it is easy to subconsciously assume that the family in front of you is a slightly different version of your own family and to interact with them accordingly. For example, with heterosexual couples in a prenatal setting, it might seem natural for the woman to be the focus of the genetic counseling session. After all, she is the one carrying the baby and the one who may undergo medical testing to assess the fetus and, if she so chooses, to elect to terminate a pregnancy. This can result in the partner taking a backseat, with his concerns and psychological and social processing marginalized. Counselors should be cognizant of the fact that couples can range comfortably from only one partner (male or female) making critical decisions to couples who wind up making decisions by a subtle back-and-forth communication process that may be invisible to the counselor but during which the counselor becomes a conduit for helpful information and perspective that aids the couple in their decision making or adaptation. Most couples have been through this process about a wide range of family issues, from the trivial to the traumatic, during their relationship.

Genetic counselors must be aware that their own preconceived notions of family and relationship can intrude on the counseling session. While you may not be comfortable in letting your spouse or partner make unilateral decisions, this can be the *modus operandi* for some couples. You do not want to impose your concept of family and family interactions on your patients. This can be particularly challenging when working with families from cultures other than your own, where the concept of a family may include in-laws, friends, former spouses, and nieces (McGrath and Edwards 2009).

While family sessions are often valued by patients and important for many of the reasons cited, a common challenge for genetic counselors is meeting the needs of young adults when their parents are in the session. A particularly tricky scenario is the diagnosis of a condition or risk in a young adult when the affected parent is in the room. While the family may have explicitly requested a joint session, they also may not have fully imagined the results they were given and may be unprepared for the collision of concerns that have been released. For this very reason, many clinics establish a policy (there does not have to be an actual policy but a decision the team made about how they offer services) that they start first with the patient alone and add the parents or other family members with time. This allows the young adult to receive the results in a more private setting and to ask the counselor questions without the constraint of being concerned about how the affected parent may feel. When you start with everyone in the room, even if you sense that the young adults are not asking the questions they may have or have gone quiet about how they are feeling, it is not impossible to ask the parents to leave the room, but it is hard and even the young adults themselves will often say, "No, they can stay." They do not want to admit even to themselves that having their affected parent present is having an effect on the interaction. As such, a policy that begins with the patient only and adds others as requested leaves open more opportunities. We have had patients get their parents immediately, and if that is their preference, it should be honored. However, cases where all family members were together at the start constituted one of the most common conundrums discussed within a peer supervision group of genetic counselors attended by one of the authors (Biesecker).

Religion and Spirituality

The majority of clients seen by genetic counselors have some degree of affiliation with an organized religion. About 70% of the US population identified as Christian in 2014 (Pew Research Fund 2015a). Worldwide, about a third of people identify as Christian, about 23% as Muslim, about 16% as unaffiliated, and about 15% as Hindu (Pew Research Fund 2015b). By and large, compared to the general population, genetic counselors are more likely to be Jewish than Christian and are less likely than their parents to believe in God, attend religious services, pray, and believe in an afterlife (Cragun et al. 2009). But most subscribe to some religious affiliation and have active and enriching spiritual lives.

Patients may not feel that it is appropriate to bring up religious issues within the context of genetic counseling, although studies on this are inconsistent (Sagaser et al. 2016; Thompson et al. 2016). Genetic counselors trained in the sciences and with a good grasp of statistics and probability may initially be confused when they hear statements from patients such as "Well, it's all in God's hands" or "I am putting my trust in God" or "God never gives us more than we can handle." However, the goal is not to separate the science from the patient's religious beliefs. For many patients, religion is a key component of their ethos, psyche, and means of understanding and relating to the world they live in. The genetic counselor should not try to steer patients away from such beliefs in the mistaken fear that patients are not understanding what is being said to them and are denying the reality of the risks or the problem at hand. This would be a significant mistake on the counselor's part.

Religious beliefs can be flexible for some clients. For example, the Catholic Church is clear about its prohibition against the willful termination of life at all stages and specifically abortion. However, it is not uncommon for Catholic patients, as well as others who subscribe to a similar religious perspective, to consider abortion when confronted with the results of diagnostic prenatal testing. In this case, genetic counselors must be sensitive to the fact that the parents are not just confronting the possible loss of their pregnancy and wished-for child, but also considering the possibility of going against a core precept of their religious faith. Some clients may find some justification for deciding to terminate their pregnancy, while others do not. Choosing to have an abortion can be a difficult and guilt-inducing process. "God is loving and forgiving, and He understands that we sometimes have to make difficult decisions based on love" is an attitude adopted by some patients to remedy the conflict between their decision and their religious precepts.

An example of genetic counseling/testing being incorporated into religious traditions with the goal of betterment of the faithful is the Dor Yeshorim program. For ultra-Orthodox Jews, arranged marriages—*shidduchim*—are common and prospective mates are selected by families or by professional matchmakers called *shadchanim*. In this tradition, the family's wealth and its health history were important factors when matching potential mates. In the Dor Yeshorim program, the marriageable population is screened for carrier status of a number of genetic diseases, many of which occur at increased frequency among Ashkenazi Jews. Although carrier status is kept confidential, a man and woman will not be matched if they happen to be carriers for the same recessive disorders. While this program is not without its critics (Raz 2009), for some ultra-Orthodox Jews this is a very acceptable practice that is consistent with their longstanding religious traditions and demonstrates the ability of even the oldest religions to continually adapt to the modern world.

Trying to dissuade patients from making religious interpretations of their situations and predicaments will only alienate patients, and both counselor and client will leave the session dissatisfied and unfulfilled. Counselors should encourage patients to express and expand on how religion helps them to better understand and cope with their circumstances as well as give psychological meaning to the experience. Consultation with pastoral services or with local religious leaders can help counselors better understand and interpret the religious context of their patients' behaviors, beliefs, and choices.

REFERENCES

Austin, S. 2010. "Developmentally Based Approaches for Counseling Children and Adolescents." In *Genetic Counseling Practice: Advanced Concepts and Skills*, edited by B. S. Leroy, P. M. Veach, and D. M. Bartels, 253–80. New York: Wiley-Blackwell.

Baldacchino, A., D. J. Balfour, F. Passetti, G. Humphris, and K. Matthews. 2012. "Neuropsychological Consequences of Chronic Opioid Use: A Quantitative Review and Meta-analysis." *Neuroscience and Biobehavioral Reviews* 36: 2056–68. doi:10.1016/j.neubiorev.2012.06.006.

Batte, B., J. P. Sheldon, P. Arscott, D. J. Huismann, L. Salberg, S. M. Day, and B. M. Yashar. 2015. "Family Communication in a Population at Risk for Hypertrophic Cardiomyopathy." *Journal of Genetic Counseling* 24: 336–48. doi:10.1007/s10897-014-9774-8.

Burke, A. L., J. L. Mathias, and L. A. Denson. 2015. "Psychological Functioning of People Living with Chronic Pain: A Meta-analytic Review." *British Journal of Clinical Psychology* 54: 345–60. doi:10.1111/bjc.12078.

Butrick, M., S. Kelly, B. N. Peshkin, G. Luta, R. Nusbaum, G. W. Hooker, . . . M.D. Schwartz. 2015. "Disparities in Uptake of BRCA1/2 Genetic Testing in a Randomized Trial of Telephone Counseling." *Genetics in Medicine* 17: 467–75. doi:10.1038/gim.2014.125.

Cáceda, R., C. B. Nemeroff, and P. D. Harvey. 2014. "Toward an Understanding of Decision Making in Severe Mental Illness." *Journal of Neuropsychiatry & Clinical Neurosciences* 26: 196–213. doi:10.1176/appi.neuropsych.12110268.

Callard, A., J. Williams, and H. Skirton. 2012. "Counseling Adolescents and the Challenges for Genetic Counselors." *Journal of Genetic Counseling* 21: 505–509. doi:10.1007/s10897-011-9460-z.

Cragun, D., D. Bonner, J. Kim, M. R. Akbari, S. A. Narod, A. Gomez-Fuego, . . . Pal T. 2015. "Factors Associated with Genetic Counseling and BRCA Testing in a Population-Based Sample of Young Black Women with Breast Cancer." *Breast Cancer Research & Treatment* 15: 169–76. doi:10.1007/s10549-015-3374-7.

Cragun, R. T., A. R. Woltanski, M. F. Myers, and D. L. Cragun. 2009. "Genetic Counselors' Religiosity and Spirituality: Are Genetic Counselors Different from the General Population?" *Journal of Genetic Counseling* 18: 551–66. doi:10.1007/s10897-009-9241-0.

Daly, B., and O. I. Olopade. 2015. "A Perfect Storm: How Tumor Biology, Genomics, and Health Care Delivery Patterns Collide to Create a Racial Survival Disparity in Breast Cancer and Proposed Interventions for Change." *CA A Cancer Journal for Clinicians* 65: 221–38. doi:10.3322/caac.21271.

Daly, M. B. 2009. "The Impact of Social Roles on the Experience of Men in BRCA1/2 Families: Implications for Counseling." *Journal of Genetic Counseling* 18: 42–48. doi:10.1007/s10897-008-9183-y.

Duncan, R. E., and M-A. Young. 2013. "Tricky Teens: Are They Really Tricky or Do Genetic Health Professionals Simply Require More Training in Adolescent Health?" *Personalized Medicine* 10: 589–600. doi.org/10.2217/pme.13.49.

Epping, E. A., J. I. Kim, D. Craufurd, T. M. Brashers-Krug, K. E. Anderson, E. McCusker E., . . . PREDICT-HD Investigators and Coordinators of the Huntington Study Group. 2016. "Longitudinal Psychiatric Symptoms in Prodromal Huntington's Disease: A Decade of Data." *American Journal of Psychiatry* 173: 184–92. doi:10.1176/appi.ajp.2015.14121551.

Evans, C. 2006. *Genetic Counselling: A Psychological Approach*. New York: Cambridge University Press. http://dx.doi.org/10.1017/CBO9780511543746.

Finlay, E., J. E. Stopfer, E. Burlingame, K. G. Evans, K. L. Nathanson, B. L. Weber, . . . S. M. Domchek. 2008. "Factors Determining Dissemination of Results and Uptake of Genetic Testing in Families with Known BRCA1/2 Mutations." *Genetic Testing* 12: 81–91. doi:10.1089/gte.2007.0037.

Flores, G., M. Abreu, C. P. Barone, R. Bachur, and H. Lin. 2012. "Errors of Medical Interpretation and Their Potential Clinical Consequences: A Comparison of Professional versus Ad Hoc versus No Interpreters." *Annals of Emergency Medicine* 60, no. 5: 545–53. doi:10.1016/j.annemergmed.2012.01.025.

Gleichgerrcht, E., A. Ibáñez, M. Roca, T. Torralva, and F. Manes. 2010. "Decision-Making Cognition in Neurodegenerative Diseases." *Nature Reviews Neurology* 6: 611–23. doi:10.1038/nrneurol.2010.148.

Glessner, H. D., E. VandenLangenberg, P. M. Veach, and B. S. LeRoy. 2012. "Are Genetic Counselors and GLBT Patients 'on the Same Page'? An Investigation of Attitudes, Practices, and Genetic Counseling Experiences." *Journal of Genetic Counseling* 21: 326–36. doi:10.1007/s10897-011-9403-8.

Graves, J. L. Jr. 2002. *The Emperor's New Clothes. Biological Theories of Race at the Millennium.* New Brunswick, NJ: Rutgers University Press.

Graves, K. D., R. Gatammah, B. N. Peshkin, A. Krieger, C. Gell, H. B. Valdimarsdottir, and M. D. Schwartz. 2011. "BRCA1/2 Genetic Testing Uptake and Psychosocial Outcomes in Men." *Familial Cancer* 10: 213–23. doi:10.1007/s10689-011-9425-2.

Henry, J. D., W. von Hippel, P. Molenberghs, T. Lee, and P. S. Sachdev. 2016. "Clinical Assessment of Social Cognitive Function in Neurological Disorders." *Nature Review Neurology* 12: 28–39. doi:10.1038/nrneurol.2015.229.

Hicks, E. M., M. S. Litwin, and S. L. Maliski. 2014. "Latino Men and Familial Risk Communication about Prostate Cancer." *Oncology Nursing Forum* 41: 509–16. doi:10.1188/14.ONF.509-516.

Hobbs, G. S., M. B. Landrum, N. K. Arora, P. A. Ganz, M. van Ryn, J. C. Weeks, . . . N. L. Keating. 2015. "The Role of Families in Decisions Regarding Cancer Treatments." *Cancer* 121: 1079–87. doi:10.1002/cncr.29064.

Hsu, C. D., X. Wang, D. V. Habif Jr., C. X. Ma, and K. J. Johnson. 2017. "Breast Cancer Stage Variation and Survival in Association with Insurance Status and Sociodemographic Factors in US Women 18 to 64 Years Old." *Cancer* 123, no. 16: 3125–31. doi:10.1002/cncr.30722.

Hunt, L. M., and K. B. de Voogd. 2007. "Are Good Intentions Good Enough? Informed Consent without Trained Interpreters." *Journal of General Internal Medicine* 22: 598–605. doi:10.1007/s11606-007-0136-1.

Ingles, J., R. Johnson, T. Sarina, L. Yeates, C. Burns, B. Gray, . . . C. Semsarian. 2015. "Social Determinants of Health in the Setting of Hypertrophic Cardiomyopathy." *International Journal of Cardiology* 184: 743–49. doi:10.1016/j.ijcard.2015.03.070.

Jeon, K. C., L. S. Chen, and P. Goodson. 2012. "Decision to Abort after a Prenatal Diagnosis of Sex Chromosome Abnormality: A Systematic Review of the Literature." *Genetics in Medicine* 14: 27–38. doi:10.1038/gim.0b013e31822e57a7.

Karliner, L. S., E. A. Jacobs, A. H. Chen, and S. Mutha. 2007. "Do Professional Interpreters Improve Clinical Care for Patients with Limited English Proficiency? A Systematic Review of the Literature." *Health Services Research* 42: 727–54.

Krugman, Paul. 2011. "Patients Are Not Consumers." *New York Times*. April 21, 2011. https://www.nytimes.com/2011/04/22/opinion/22krugman.html.

Lakes, K. D., E. Vaughan, M. Jones, W. Burke, D. Baker, and J. M. Swanson. 2012. "Diverse Perceptions of the Informed Consent Process: Implications for the Recruitment and Participation of Diverse Communities in the National Children's Study." *American Journal of Community Psychology* 49, no. 1–2: 215–32. doi:10.1007/s10464-011-9450-1.

Lobb, E. A., C. L. Gaff, B. Meiser, P. N. Butow, R. Osseiran-Moisson, and N. Hallowell. 2009. "Attendance of Men at the Familial Cancer Clinic: What They Value from the Consultation." *Genetics in Medicine* 11: 434–40. doi:10.1038/sj.bjc.6601502.

Makadon, H. J. 2011. "Ending LGBT Invisibility in Health Care: The First Step in Ensuring Equitable Care." *Cleveland Clinic Journal of Medicine* 78: 220–24. doi:10.3949/ccjm.78gr.10006.

McCalman, J., C. Jongen, and R. Bainbridge. 2017. "Organisational Systems' Approaches to Improving Cultural Competence in Healthcare: A Systematic Scoping Review of the Literature." *International Journal of Equity in Health* 16, no. 1: 78. doi:10.1186/s12939-017-0571-5.

McGrath, B. B., and K. L. Edwards. 2009. "When Family Means More (or Less) than Genetics: The Intersection of Culture, Family and Genomics." *Journal of Transcultural Nursing* 20: 270–77. doi:10.1177/1043659609334931.

Mittman, I. S., J. V. Bowie, and S. Maman. 2007. "Exploring the Discourse between Genetic Counselors and Orthodox Jewish Community Members Related to Reproductive Genetic Technology." *Patient Education and Counseling* 65: 230–36.

Montgomery, S. V., A. M. Barsevick, B. L. Egleston, R. Bingler, K. Ruth, S. M. Miller, . . . Daly MB. 2013. "Preparing Individuals to Communicate Genetic Test Results to Their Relatives: Report of a Randomized Control Trial." *Familial Cancer* 12, no. 3: 537–46. doi:10.1007/s10689-013-9609-z.

Moore, H. C. 2014. "An Overview of Chemotherapy-Related Cognitive Dysfunction, or 'Chemobrain.'" *Oncology* 28: 797–804.

Nápoles, A. M., J. Santoyo-Olsson, L. S. Karliner, S. E. Gregorich, and E. J. Pérez-Stable. 2015. "Inaccurate Language Interpretation and Its Clinical Significance in the Medical Encounters of Spanish-Speaking Latinos." *Medical Care* 53: 940–47. doi:10.1097/MLR.0000000000000422.

National Society of Genetic Counselors. 2018. Professional Status Survey. https://www.nsgc.org/p/do/sd/sid=7524.

Office for Civil Rights Policy Guidance. n.d. "Title VI Prohibition Against National Origin Discrimination as It Affects Persons with Limited English Proficiency." Office for Civil Rights, U S Department of Health and Human Services [cited 2016, June 19]. http://www.hhs.gov/civil-rights/for-providers/laws-regulations-guidance/guidance-federal-financial-assistance-title-VI/index.html.

Paulsen, J. S., M. M. Smith, J. D. Long; PREDICT HD investigators and Coordinators of the Huntington Study Group. 2013. "Cognitive Decline in Prodromal Huntington Disease: Implications for Clinical Trials." *Journal of Neurology, Neurosurgery, and Psychiatry* 84: 1233–39. doi:10.1136/jnnp-2013-305114.

Pew Research Fund. 2015a. *America's Changing Religious Landscape.* http://www.pewforum.org/2015/05/12/americas-changing-religious-landscape/.

Pew Research Fund. 2015b. *The Future of World Religions: Population Growth Projections, 2010–2050.* http://www.pewforum.org/2015/04/02/religious-projections-2010-2050/.

Pinkhasov, R. M., J. Wong, J. Kashanian, M. Lee, D. B. Samadi, M. M. Pinkhasov, and R. Shabsigh. 2010. "Are Men Shortchanged on Health? Perspective on Health Care Utilization and Health Risk Behavior in Men and Women in the United States." *International Journal of Clinical Practice* 64: 475–87. doi:10.1111/j.1742-1241.2009.02290.x.

Preloran, H. M., C. H. Browner, and E. Lieber. 2005. "Impact of Interpreters' Approach on Latinas' Use of Amniocentesis." *Health Education & Behavior* 32: 599–612. doi:10.1177/1090198105278745.

Raymond, C. W. 2014. "Conveying Information in the Interpreter-Mediated Medical Visit: The Case of Epistemic Brokering." *Patient Education & Counseling* 97: 38–46. doi:10.1016/j.pec.2014.05.020.

Raz, A. E. 2009. "Can Population-Based Carrier Screening Be Left to the Community?" *Journal of Genetic Counseling* 18: 114–18. doi:10.1007/s10897-008-9209-5.

Sagaser, K. G., S. Shahrukh Hashmi, R. D. Carter, J. Lemons, H. Mendez-Figueroa, S. Nassef, . . . C. N. Singletary. 2016. "Spiritual Exploration in the Prenatal Genetic Counseling Session." *Journal of Genetic Counseling* 25, no. 5: 923–35. doi:10.1007/s10897-015-9920-y.

Schaa, K. L., D. L. Roter, B. B. Biesecker, L. A. Cooper, and L. H. Erby. 2015. "Genetic Counselors' Implicit Racial Attitudes and Their Relationship to Communication." *Health Psychology* 34: 111–19. doi:10.1037/hea0000155.

Sharaf, R. N., P. Myer, C. D. Stave, L. C. Diamond, and U. Ladabaum. 2013. "Uptake of Genetic Testing by Relatives of Lynch Syndrome Probands: A Systematic Review." *Clinical Gastroenterology and Hepatology* 11: 1093–100. doi:10.1016/j.cgh.2013.04.044.

Sheppard, V. B., D. Mays, T. LaVeist, and K. P. Tercyak. 2013. "Medical Mistrust Influences Black Women's Level of Engagement in BRCA 1/2 Genetic Counseling and Testing." *Journal of the National Medical Association* 105: 17–22.

Shiloh, S., E. Dagan, I. Friedman, N. Blank, and E. Friedman. 2013. "A Follow-up Study on Men Tested for BRCA1/BRCA2 Mutations: Impacts and Coping Processes." *Psychooncology* 22, no. 2: 417–25. doi:10.1002/pon.2106.

Strømsvik, N., M. Råheim, and E. Gjengedal. 2011. "Cancer Worry among Norwegian Male BRCA1/2 Mutation Carriers." *Familial Cancer* 10: 597–603. doi:10.1007/s10689-011-9456-8.

Strømsvik, N., M. Råheim, N. Oyen, L. F. Engebretsen, and E. Gjengedal. 2010. "Stigmatization and Male Identity: Norwegian Males' Experience after Identification as BRCA1/2 Mutation Carriers." *Journal of Genetic Counseling* 19: 360–70. doi:10.1007/s10897-010-9293-1.

Strømsvik, N., M. Råheim, N. Oyen, and E. Gjengedal. 2009. "Men in the Women's World of Hereditary Breast and Ovarian Cancer—a Systematic Review." *Familial Cancer* 8: 221–29. doi:10.1007/s10689-009-9232-1.

Sullivan, J., and A. McConkie-Rosell. 2010. "Helping Parents to Talk to Their Children." In *Family Communication About Genetics: Theory and Practice*, edited by C. L. Gaff and C. L. Bylund, 227–42. New York: Oxford University Press.

Szybowska, M., S. Hewson, B. Antle, and R. Babul-Hirji. 2007. "Assessing the Informational Needs of Adolescents with a Genetic Condition: What Do They Want to Know?" *Journal of Genetic Counseling* 16: 201–10.

Templeton, A. R. 2013. "Biological Races in Humans." *Studies in History and Philosophy of Biology Biomedical Sciences* 44, no. 3: 262–71. doi:10.1016/j.shpsc.2013.04.010.

Tercyak, K. P., editor. 2010. *Handbook of Genomics and the Family: Psychosocial Context for Children and Adolescents*. New York: Springer.

Thompson, A. B., D. Cragun, J. E. Sumerau, R. T. Cragun, V. De Gifis, and A. Trepanier. 2016. "'Be Prepared if I Bring It Up': Patients' Perceptions of the Utility of Religious and Spiritual Discussion during Genetic Counseling." *Journal of Genetic Counseling* 25, no. 5: 945–56. doi:10.1007/s10897-015-9922-9.

VandenLangenberg, E., P. M. Veach, B. S. LeRoy, and H. D. Glessner. 2012. "Gay, Lesbian, and Bisexual Patients' Recommendations for Genetic Counselors: A Qualitative Investigation." *Journal of Genetic Counseling* 21: 741–47. doi:10.1007/s10897-012-9499-5.

Vu, M., A. Azmat, T. Radejko, and A. I. Padela. 2016. "Predictors of Delayed Healthcare Seeking among American Muslim Women." *Journal of Women's Health* 25, no. 6: 586–93. doi:10.1089/jwh.2015.5517.

Weil, J. 2000. *Psychosocial Genetic Counseling*. New York: Oxford University Press.

Williams, D. R., S. A. Mohammed, J. Leavell, and C. Collins. 2010. "Race, Socioeconomic Status, and Health: Complexities, Ongoing Challenges, and Research Opportunities." *Annals of the New York Academy of Sciences* 1186: 69–101.

CHAPTER 5

Characteristics of Genetic Counselors

Perhaps the most notable characteristic of the profession of genetic counseling is the overwhelming majority of white female counselors (https://www.nsgc.org/p/cm/ld/fid=68). The genetic counseling workforce has never been broadly diverse and fails to represent the socio-ethnocultural range of clients described in Chapter 4. As a largely female profession, this leaves the men a decided minority; as such, it is challenging to know in what ways their characteristics, biases, and beliefs related to genetic counseling may differ. Some traits are likely similar to those of the women, such as those that also drew men to the profession, but others may not be (Chen et al. 2017). In this chapter, we describe the variety of traits, values, beliefs, and experiences genetic counselors bring to our challenging but rewarding clinical work.

CHARACTER TRAITS

Genetic counselors share character traits that drew them to the profession. These include high intelligence, based on the standards and selectivity of relatively small graduate programs, and scientifically minded, based on the required coursework. As found among geneticists (Geller, Tambor, and Chase 1993), genetic counselors are likely to have higher tolerance for uncertainty, as much of the information we convey to clients is probabilistic, unknown, and ambiguous (Han et al. 2011).

Counselors are also very likely to have high emotional intelligence—the ability to handle interpersonal relationships judiciously and empathically. This trait facilitates sensitivities to others and understanding of clients, contributing to counselors' ability to experience and convey empathy. Similarly, counselors are often high in dispositional optimism that facilitates their ability to see hope in the future of their clients' lives (Injeyan et al. 2011). This positive bias, balanced with realistic expectations for a wide variety of clients, reflects what is heartening and steadfast about genetic counselors. Such optimism buffers counselors somewhat from the pain and suffering of our patients and allows us to see benefits of our work exemplified in the resilience of people in difficult circumstances (Injeyan et al. 2011).

While all these traits are important assets to the practice, counseling skills still need to be developed and honed to maximize these traits as assets in caring for clients and for oneself. They can also present obstacles to care. Clients have a spectrum of tolerance for uncertainty, and those with less tolerance for uncertainty, who differ from us, may be more challenging to help. This example may be particularly prevalent given the number of uncertain test results returned to clients.

Counselors often refer to themselves socially as "control freaks." This perception likely comes from the self-awareness that they value personal control. It is no surprise that learning genetics resonated with us. It was alluring in that it made it possible to understand and predict how genetic conditions occur and where risks arise. The satisfying nature of this information resides in the attraction of the theoretical ability to control one's future. Sharing that control with patients is consistent with our preference for being in control and having choices. As such, we are more likely to encounter challenges when working to help clients who are less interested in control or who have little control over their circumstances. We need to recognize our preference for control and how it enters into our interactions with clients to ensure that our messages are congruent with their values and beliefs, and not reflections of our own preferences.

Counselors genuinely respect and value their clients. Most counselors are curious to understand them and their circumstances with the intent to use what they learn to help the clients reach their counseling goals. It is a privileged opportunity to engage in a clinical relationship with a stranger and to discuss personally meaningful and challenging issues related to health and disease, family and self. Without a high level of commitment to learning about a stranger and personalizing the interactions, genetic counseling would be at risk to become routine, leading to disengagement and disappointment.

COUNSELOR VALUES AND BELIEFS

Individuals drawn to a career in genetic counseling value the lives of disabled adults and children (Madeo et al. 2011), support reproductive freedoms (National Society of Genetic Counselors n.d.), believe those at genetic risk should not be discriminated against, and that access to health care is a universal right. Statements to these effects have been endorsed by the National Society of Genetic Counselors (https://www.nsgc.org/p/cm/ld/fid=12; https://www.nsgc.org/p/bl/et/blogaid=1007). The very practice of genetic counseling exploits clients' rights by offering options to avoid, mitigate, or treat conditions at birth, adult-onset genetic conditions, or other health threats. Support of these values and human rights is consistent with the professional practice of genetic counseling in effectively realizing its goals. Yet not all genetic counselors may support these rights. Those counselors who hold differing values and beliefs still find opportunities to support and counsel patients facing decisions they may not fully endorse (Madeo et al. 2011). This ability stems from a commitment to respect patients' preferences, facilitate informed choice, and practice a client-centered approach to care.

Within these moral and political beliefs lie genetic counselors' regard for their clients that guides how we engage with them. Most, although not all, genetic counseling clients are mentally healthy and face a potential genetic threat or have been offered a test to learn more about their health status or risks to their fetus. Even adult clients affected with a condition, assuming they are cognitively capacitated, are usually psychologically sound and have the resources to make informed decisions that align with their values and beliefs. Importantly, counselors recognize clients as capable decision makers mastering the challenges of living with their conditions.

Clients can generally articulate their views and preferences, make hard decisions for themselves, recognize their personal strengths and challenges, and, when affected or parenting an affected child, find personal strength under even very challenging circumstances and, remarkably, adapt over time. Through respect and genuineness counselors work to help clients tap into these resources.

The relationship between counselor and client is a partnership centered on the client's needs and directed by the counselor to achieve them. When clients' assets are limited due to a condition, such as one associated with lower cognitive capacity, or psychiatric illness, genetic counselors find creative ways to engage in innovative approaches to help clients make good decisions for themselves. In these cases, it may include relying on social resources such as family and community.

PERSONAL BELIEFS

Genetic counselors hold personal beliefs about the inherent ability of clients to make good decisions for themselves and benefit from learning personal genetic information. Not all of our clients meet our expectations or use information in ways that are useful or informed, but we generally credit them with the potential to do so. Genetic counselors' belief in our clients extends to their desire to become empowered to make good decisions on behalf of themselves and their families (Kessler 1999; McAllister and Dearing 2015; McAllister et al. 2008). Among counselors broadly, there is a deep respect for clients from all backgrounds and experiences who, even in the face of adversity, reveal capacities to help themselves and a willingness to engage and accept help in partnership with us.

Ethicists and scholars have described genetic counseling practice as value-free (Gervais 1993). By this, it seems they mean that counselors prioritize the primacy of clients making their own decisions aligned with their personal beliefs, a practice that may be described as promoting client preferences or upholding preference-based decision making. Yet, when we consider the array of values and beliefs that are prevalent among genetic counselors, it seems nonsensical to refer to it as value-neutral care (Rentmeester 2001). Indeed, genetic counseling involves some of the most challenging value-laden decisions people ever make: for example, whether to continue a pregnancy when a fetus is found to be affected, whether to have more biological children when there is an increased risk for a serious condition, whether to enroll one's child in a clinical trial, and whether to have genetic testing when you face a 50% risk for a neurodegenerative condition. In addition to the client-centered values inherent to these decisions are the values genetic counselors hold. Paramount is the value that what the client perceives as most important and should drive his or her decision making. Clarifying clients' values and helping clients to engage them is at the core of client-centered care.

Perhaps above all, genetic counselors value science. We were attracted to genetic counseling because genetics is fascinating; otherwise, many of us likely would have trained as clinical psychologists, or other helping professionals. And as such, we are generally enthusiastic about sharing what we favor about genetics, and how it offers clients choices they may benefit from. We are at times so enthusiastic about the science of genomics that often we slip into an interaction with clients where we dominate the session with a genetics lecture, without regard for whether our clients are engaged or benefiting from the lesson. Not everyone loves genetics the way counselors do! Most people find the terms "DNA" and "chromosomes" obscure or off-putting (Joseph et al. 2017). Dominanting sessions with genetics lectures often leave clients perplexed. They may ask themselves, "What do these words 'chromosomes' and 'DNA' have to do with my relatives?" "What does this mean about whether my daughter is getting worse?" Despite good will and intentions, genetic counselors often inundate their clients with information and alienating them, and failing to equip them to partner in the discussion. At its worst, this practice can disparage clients who do not grasp the concepts and have little idea what the counselor is explaining, leaving them humiliated or embarrassed and unlikely to speak up and say, "I don't get it." Clients rarely admit to counselors that they have been left behind in the "conversation" and rate their satisfaction with the service as high (Buchanan et al. 2015; Nieuwhof, Birnie, and van den Berg 2017; Otten et al. 2015). This may be partially due to clients' appreciation for the time and effort the counselor devoted to their concerns and the warmth most counselors exude. But the aims of counseling are not to be appreciated, but rather to help empower our clients with information and recognition of their personal resources to manage the health threat addressed in genetic counseling. As such, not only is the educational component thwarted by oversharing our appreciation for genetics, but also a therapeutic alliance between counselor and client.

There is insufficient evidence to explain why genetic counselors lecture on genetics to their patients. One theory is that it is a sharing of what we highly value. Given the intelligence, positivity, and generosity of genetic counselors, a reasonable explanation for these lectures is our desire to share something we value with others who may benefit from it, reflecting how much we favor genetics information personally and professionally. Unfortunately, this approach runs counter to how adults learn new, complex, and high-literacy information that they may have limited ways to relate to. We are naive about how hard it is for many clients to learn the science as taught. Certainly, the objective of genetic counseling to help clients and families learn genetic information to make informed choices and understand what has befallen their family flows from the practice definition (Resta et al. 2006). Yet the approach to education is lacking. We raise the issue here because the consistency with which counselors unleash a deluge of technical information on their clients suggests that this practice has more to do with who genetic counselors are than their clients' needs or session goals (Roter et al. 2006). The intention is genuine and admirable, but the execution does not serve our clients well (Ellington et al. 2011; Farrelly et al. 2012; Joseph et al. 2017).

PATIENT EDUCATORS

Importantly, genetic counselors believe in clients' abilities to represent and care for themselves and to make informed choices for themselves and their families. We respect and admire our clients, and that goes a long way toward working to establish a therapeutic relationship. Genuinely conveying this respect early in the relationship is a key step toward winning clients' trust and openness to engaging in a partnership to assess and use genetic information in their lives. This belief reflects a strong intent of genetic counseling.

Further, genetic counselors believe that our clients can learn a sufficient amount of genetic information to use it effectively in their lives. The decisions clients make based on the information may not result in reduction of the incidence of those living with genetic conditions but should reflect well-considered value-based decision making—clients executing their agency. Due to our belief in the central role of genetic information in empowering clients, we need to ensure that how we educate our clients is effective in their mastery of key or essential information. For our highly educated and intelligent patients, it may be straightforward to enhance or adjust what they already know or believe about inheritance or choices. But many clients are not scientifically or health literate, so the ways we educate them have to be tailored. Partnering with clients so they feel safe and comfortable discussing what they understand and what they do not is critical to the endeavor (Joseph et al. 2017). A client's expressed desire to learn makes it much more likely that the exchange with a genetic counselor will be effective in teaching essential information. The genetic counselor can target exchange of desired information accordingly. The challenge of genetics education is in determining what a reasonable and useful amount of information is for a specific client, as what is appropriate for one may not be for another. For example, while some clients may readily understand the concept of chromosomes and a description of nondisjunction as the cause of a prenatal diagnosis, others may find a more general description to be sufficient for their learning needs; say, that a developing baby can have too much or too little information that determines how it grows and develops.

In our enthusiasm about the science to empower our clients, genetic counselors tend to make assumptions about clients' needs, styles of learning, and priorities. Providers may assume first-time clients are naive to genetics or likely to have misinformation they learned on the internet or from relatives. Perhaps it is such assumptions that propel genetic counselors to provide the information they perceive their clients need (Joseph et al. 2019). Studies show that genetic counselors tend to routinize their information delivery and counseling approach (Ellington et al. 2006; Farrelly et al. 2012; Joseph et al. 2017). We need to resist the strong effect of our assumptions about what our clients will choose to do or even about what they need. Otherwise we will play a more direct role in the client's decision making than we intend (Ubel, Scherr, and Fagerlin 2018). For example, asking, "Do you want to know X?" is not a useful question. Most clients are likely to answer "yes" to this question. They do not want to miss anything they should know or be provided less information than others. Being naive about their circumstances is what they fear. Clients value knowledge as a perceived way to find control. In asking this well-intentioned question, a pattern of communicating can result in which the counselor asks, the client replies "yes," and information is provided. Then the counselor asks whether the client wants to know about Y, and the cycle continues. This fails as a shared learning process where the client gains new information built on prior understanding and becomes sufficiently knowledgeable to ask specific questions to further expand understanding of his or her health risks.

Similarly, when clients express their desire to "know everything they can" about their child's condition, for example, providers often take this literally. Yet if they first paused to ask clients what they understand about their circumstances and what they would like to know, counselors could weave new information into clients' existing knowledge and frame of reference. Parents' expertise with their child's condition and/or the family history of a condition can be exploited in educating clients, as they have experience counselors often don't. When counselors do explore what clients already know, some clients may feel hesitant to respond; they may fear misusing genetic or medical terms or feel anxious that they will "get it wrong" in the presence of a professional. If counselors can gently coax clients into sharing by reassuring them that they are not being judged, most people will try to describe what they understand, and what they imagine or fear may happen to their child. Learning clients' understanding and expectations often reveals their cognitions or "mental models" for the condition and how it occurred. New information about the cause and risks can be more readily learned when it is integrated into existing cognitive models, and later put to good use.

When clients are uninformed or misinformed about the risk or condition in their family, they may feel more vulnerable in their relationship with the counselor. As the counselor imparts information that is novel or conflicts with clients' understanding, they may feel less in control and poorly understood. These affective responses can lead to a distancing from the counselor. Counselors need to attend to the beliefs of the client prior to working to dispel them out of respect and the need to understand how those beliefs provide an explanation that makes sense in the family. Counselors should not forgo an opportunity to assess client knowledge and beliefs prior to sharing what they know. Considerations include how much information clients can absorb, the relative value of the information, respect for the ways people make meaning of information, the ability of clients to hold multiple causal attributions, how relatable the technical jargon is, and the sociocultural context into which the information is delivered (Joseph et al. 2017). The needs of the client and the context should serve as guidance for the counselor in delivering client-centered information in a way that addresses what the client has come to understand.

Counselors respect the central role clients play in assessing and managing genetic information. They theoretically grant their clients agency in determining what is of value to them and important in making informed preference-based decisions. Yet certain information is medically recommended, such as screening for those at higher risk for a disease. In these situations, counselors advocate a course of action and work with clients to assume responsibility and willingness to follow up, as it is in their best interest to preserve their health. Issuing health screening recommendations is often quite directive. Some counselors advocate for the use of motivational interviewing techniques to achieve positive client outcomes (Ash 2017). While conveying the information about increased risk is important, igniting motivations to follow up on these recommendations is essential to achieving reduced morbidity and mortality; merely conveying risk information is insufficient (Fagerlin, Zikmund-Fisher, and Ubel 2011). Counselors may hold beliefs that accurate understanding of risk will lead to engagement in recommended health behaviors, but they also appreciate that one does not guarantee the other. Clients often do not perceive risks accurately. Coupled with this challenge, a number of variables and practical barriers play a role in whether patients will pursue recommended medical care. How clients perceive risk and assess the facilitators and barriers to acting on it varies. Here we emphasize that counselors' beliefs about the value of risk information may differ from the ways that it is perceived and used by clients.

Adult education research indicates that clients are not likely to be able to learn and remember more than three to five new concepts during one interaction, no matter how capable, motivated, or engaged clients are (Cowan 2010). New information is laid down by adults in relation to what they already know and what they are seeking to learn (Miller and Stoeckel 2017). The client's mental model, or explanation for the risk or circumstance, is critical to the counselor's delivery of new information that may support current understanding, refute it, or have no relation to it at all. In the latter case, new information is not likely to be retained. Effective adult education is based on appreciation for different learning styles as proposed by Kolb: abstract (thinking), concrete (feeling), active (doing), and reflective (watching) (https://www.simplypsychology.org/learning-kolb.html). Experiential learning theory applies to clients as they often present having had an experience that led to a readiness to learn that facilitates their ability to take on novel information, such as having an affected family member or receiving a prenatal screening result. Educating our clients happens within a deliberate partnership by which the educator and the learner work to understand the foundation on which new information is built. The learner comes to understand that he or she may not have the full story, only a single story or an angle to the story that does not fully explain the circumstances, and come to recognize a need to know new or different information.

For teaching to be effective, the genetic counselor needs to break down the essential new information into understandable chunks or units that stand alone and can be related to one another as the exchange advances. Further, scientific or technical language needs to be minimized. For example, teaching DNA and chromosomes in most cases is not necessary to convey patterns of inheritance. Studies on the public's understanding of genetics suggest that most people understand that traits and disease can run in families (Condit 2010). For clients who have no conceptual understanding of a cell, it is wise to avoid discussing cellular structures. Yet, teaching inheritance patterns is important in genetic counseling, and many of us seem to believe that to empower our clients, we need to apprise them of the constitution of a gene and where it resides. This approach can derail clients from learning basic concepts such as recurrence risks when it includes detail for which they have no reference. A more productive approach is to understand how a client makes sense of the risks based on family and medical history. These perceptions may not follow scientific logic, but relating new information to beliefs already held is the most promising approach for clients to learn. Much of the information we convey is theoretical in that it predicts future possibilities, and to understand this requires proficiency in abstract thinking. For more educated clients, this is not difficult, but clients with less education or those who are cognitively challenged can find it very difficult; probabilities may need to be made concrete.

While belief in our clients' abilities is paramount and appropriate, we cannot assume that clients learn similarly or desire or can use the same information. Tailoring information delivery to the client's learning style and needs is of utmost importance to achieving understanding. A wide range exists in what clients come in already knowing, and when the client knows very little, the counselor needs to be creative in exploring what the client does know that can be linked to teaching new information. Further, evidence shows that use of teach-back methods helps clients to retain what they learn and allows counselors to assess whether the client has mastered essential information (Fagerlin et al. 2011) (https://www.ahrq.gov/professionals/quality-patient-safety/quality-resources/tools/literacy-toolkit/healthlittoolkit2-tool5.html). These are valuable techniques that can be used to check understanding without quizzing patients and making them feel self-conscious. Partnering as teacher and learner to openly address what the client understands is as important to effective education as it is to the reciprocal exchanges in relational counseling described in Chapter 8.

Ultimately, the success of client education depends in large measure on the effectiveness of the counselor at communicating pertinent information in the context of what the client knows and seeks, and the client's style and capacity to learn it. The expertise of genetic counselors as educators depends on their familiarity with education theories, adult learning, and health communication. Any genetic counselor who leans heavily on an educational practice model should use one that is built on evidence of how adults learn. Genetic counselors may benefit from advanced training in health communication to understand strategies and barriers to effective education of health-related information.

COUNSELOR BIASES

In parallel with training in genetics, counselors tend to believe that the essence of client decision making depends on the underlying science. And yet, cognitive beliefs and affective responses to the scientific information drive client decision making in complex ways. We concur that science should be at the core, but the ways clients interpret and react to that information lead to health outcomes (Ferrer, Klein, and Graff 2017; French, Cameron, and Benton 2017). As such, genetic counselors need to recognize their bias toward achieving "accurate" client understanding—that is, the same understanding as the counselor. While counselors would rightly not settle for knowing clients were making decisions based on misinformation, we do need to appreciate that how clients make meaning of information can seem illogical to us. It may not meet our expectations for a "rational" understanding yet may be predictable based on the ways that people make decisions in the context of uncertainty (Ariely 2009). Counselors' awareness of their bias in this regard is key to respecting clients' perceptions and their "predictable irrationality."

Counselors may also have a strong negative bias toward withholding information—perhaps due to concerns that an incomplete lesson in genetics could be viewed as inadequate or judged as "poor" genetics education and counseling. Genetic counselors instead should feel confident in their efforts to tailor information and parse out the essential bits for their clients. If effectively done, clients can build on the information over time. Evidence supports this approach as most effective in meeting clients' needs (Ubel et al. 2018).

COMPASSION FATIGUE

Several studies of genetic counselors reveal self-reports of compassion fatigue (Injeyan et al. 2011; Udipi, McCarthy Veach, and LeRoy 2008; Werner-Lin, McCoyd, and Bernhardt 2016). This is generally defined as the depletion that can arise among practitioners caring for patients with debilitating conditions. It speaks to a lack of energy to invest in others and has been described as an acute and intense process (Benoit, McCarthy Veach, and LeRoy 2007). Remarkably, genetic counselors self-report significant rates of compassion fatigue, despite their generally optimistic and hopeful dispositions and high ratings of satisfaction in their work (Injeyan et al. 2011; Werner-Lin et al. 2016). Sources of compassion fatigue are reported as working with patients with untreatable conditions, having busy jobs with seemingly limitless responsibilities, and a strong desire to help others that can result in cost to ourselves (Benoit et al. 2007). Benoit and colleagues suggest that counselors engage in coping strategies such as disengagement from patient suffering. Sahhar and colleagues (2008) wrote a reply suggesting that disengagement can be counterproductive for counselors and can lower, rather than enhance, feelings of empathy for clients. They added that compassion fatigue may be explained somewhat by countertransference and argued for the importance of peer supervision to understand when it may be occurring.

Compassion fatigue has been discussed as a significant issue for genetic counselors but one that may be amenable to interventions (Injeyan et al. 2011). Silver and colleagues (2018) conducted a study of 441 genetic counselors involved in direct patient care that yielded results on the use of mindfulness activities in significantly increasing work engagement and empathy. The investigators argued that mindfulness practices may prevent compassion fatigue and serve as a means for recovery.

Professional burnout is a distinct but overlapping concept with compassion fatigue. The former is generally a longer-term process that has many causes, primarily not those directly related to patient interactions. In the 2011 study of 355 genetic counselors by Injeyan and colleagues, burnout was the strongest correlate with compassion fatigue. Both of these negative consequences of empathy expressed by caring professionals can lead practitioners to leave the field.

For counselors who experience compassion fatigue or burnout, self-care is of prime importance. Supervision provides an opportunity to explore the effects of one's casework on one's personal well-being, and to gain insights and strength from peer support. Further, counselors benefit from regular exercise and time spent away from work. For those experiencing exhaustion or negative affect, psychotherapy may help counselors identify the sources that may lead to compassion burnout. Prevention of negative consequences of genetic counseling includes making the effort to approach each case as a new opportunity to learn about a person who can be helped to find his or her cognitive and affective strengths and personal and social resources. Further, taking note of one's connection to patients, success in providing good care, and personal and professional growth also contributes to making the work sustaining.

Genetic counseling practice is made more challenging with clients who come from a different socio-ethnocultural group than the counselor. Yet these clients can be assisted to effectively engage in genetic counseling. A key attribute to making this happen is for the counselor to be keenly aware of cultural and social discrepancies between the counselor's background and the client's. How enculturated is the client into US health-related beliefs and health-care systems? From the start, learning about clients' personal medical beliefs and expectations of counseling is important to arriving at mutually understood goals. Counselors' awareness of their own assumptions or biases toward people who differ from them in background and ethnocultural group is of the utmost importance (see the discussion of implicit bias in Chapter 4). It can help to discuss strategies with peers in supervision and to attend to the ways we may be diminished when our efforts are less successful with less familiar types of clients.

SELF-KNOWLEDGE

Prior to learning about our clients, we need to know ourselves well (Kessler 1992). As a graduate student, you likely already know a great deal about yourself. What we mean by self-awareness is your ability in a counseling relationship to understand how your personal traits, in conjunction with your clinical skills, affect your clients, and how your clients, in turn, affect you. Self-awareness includes, among other examples, understanding your traits and how they interface with those of others, your reactions to learning private and emotionally charged information about a stranger, what may upset or concern you when witnessed, and how or when you may be most tempted to respond to a client as though he or she were a friend or relative because of how familiar he or she feels. To counsel clients, you need to understand yourself thoroughly. In addition to knowing about your disposition and personality, there are experiences counselors have had with others—family members, friends, and past clients—that affect how we interact with patients. Past experiences certainly can be used to inform your counseling and enhance your skills, but this is best accomplished with professional guidance. A counseling supervisor or therapist can help genetic counselors understand when and how they may be projecting their own needs onto a client or responding to a patient based on personal experience or expectations rather than responding in the client's best interests. These can be hard to detect in one's own work, thus the value of a skilled third party.

In no way does the need for self-awareness imply that genetic counselors are more prone to psychological struggles than other helping professionals. It is human to respond to others as we would like people to respond to us and as others have responded to us in the past. However, we need to be aware of our unique nature so that we can be alert to when our responses to clients may be interfering with or distracting us from our work to the detriment of our clients, and when the work may be challenging our limits and negatively affecting our well-being.

Students in clinical psychology graduate programs are required to be in psychotherapy during their training. Knowing oneself is regarded as critical to becoming a healthy and effective counselor or therapist. Genetic counseling programs differ in that students have no such requirements. Yet all caring professionals benefit from self-awareness and the expertise of a therapist in helping us understand ourselves in relationship to our clients. The use of counseling support services or professional supervision during genetic counseling training should be embraced as students learn to navigate the interactions they have with clients in challenging circumstances. Most of us are relatively blind to our shortcomings, biases, and needs and would benefit from the insights of a skilled therapist to become further self-aware and learn to monitor and contain them in caring for others.

All of us have sensitivities when clients remind us of something about ourselves or valued others—areas potent for countertransference (Hyatt 2012; Kessler 1992; Likhite 2000; Reeder et al. 2017). This is when the counseling veers into addressing our own needs in the guise of helping our clients. The counselor may transfer thoughts and feelings about someone else or about oneself onto the client and respond to the client accordingly. Generally, this goes on below one's awareness and typically it is not a productive experience for the counselor or the client. Further, it reflects a lack of awareness about when and how we may be vulnerable to countertransference. Addressing these areas with colleagues or a therapist is important for self-care and to providing excellent patient care. Self-exploration in professional supervision can help counselors develop their self-awareness over the course of their career and learn how topics or circumstances that provoke countertransference may evolve over one's lifetime. When one has young children, for instance, issues in pediatrics may inform our counseling but also interfere with our effectiveness. Awareness of this dynamic process may help reinforce the importance of longitudinal commitment to supervision and/or psychotherapy.

Dr. Seymour Kessler, while conducting workshops with genetic counseling graduate students, would emphasize the importance of audio-recording one's cases, discussing them in professional supervision, reflecting on them privately, and writing out partial transcripts for deeper reflection on the interactions. Dr. Kessler often reminded the students that "counselors recall their cases as they hope that they went or as they fear that they went, but never as they actually went." For this reason, returning to the case transcript is exceedingly valuable, not only in graduate school but throughout one's career.

In our experience, the majority of clients agree to having their clinic visits recorded for professional supervision and often comment that they are fine with the idea that their case may be an asset to a student's training or that their counselor continues to work on his or her professional skills. The Johns Hopkins University/National Human Genome Research Institute genetic counseling program requires genetic counseling students to record their cases for assessment in professional supervision. When the program originated, supervisors resisted students asking patients to record cases as it differed from how they were trained. But over time, they came to see the benefits (such as when they, the supervisors, left the room and a client revealed something important to the student that was captured on the audiotape, or when they could return to a portion of the case that the student recalled differently than they did). Almost all supervisors and training sites agree to this practice of recording casework. Students share the digital recordings weekly in supervision with a professional supervisor. They may chose to discuss portions that went well or went less well and discuss why and how their work related to their case goals. The supervisor keeps in mind how the skills discussed demonstrate progress in reaching the students' longitudinal learning goals.

Clinical supervision occurs in every graduate program and serves as the primary source for learning clinical skills from direct work with patients and clients, coupled with the feedback and guidance from the onsite supervisor. Professional supervision differs considerably from this clinical work. Out of respect for clinical supervisors and their expertise, graduate faculty recognize that they often do not have the expertise to offer clinical feedback on cases. They may not work in the institute and may not fully understand the goals and protocols in the center, so they relinquish specific case guidance to the onsite supervisors. Similarly, the clinical supervisors often lack knowledge of the students' overall progress in their graduate education, and where they are in learning to establish therapeutic relationships with their clients. Longer-term goals can be subsumed within professional supervision where students reflect on their casework as it represents progression through stages of relationship building with clients. For example, a student may be very consistent in assessing client needs, using open-ended questions to learn what clients understand about their situation and what concerns they have. The student may be working on using clarifications and paraphrases to understand client thinking and reflection of feelings to capture affect. These are key aspects to establishing a therapeutic relationship (discussed in Chapter 8). Professional supervision can be a tremendous asset to learning these skills and awakening students to what worked in advancing the relationship and what was less effective and why. This is where the process may be more about learning who we are in relation to our clients and what we bring with us into those relationships.

At the time this text was written, only one other US genetic counseling graduate program, at the University of California at Stanislaw, used audiotaping for professional supervision. To witness the tremendous strides that students achieve learning about themselves in relation to their clients in this way makes it difficult to envision how students would otherwise gain sufficient insight and grow from feedback that facilitates learning how to be in a healthy and helpful relationship with clients. Professional supervision in graduate training can be viewed as the start of supervision as a career-long pursuit and may lead some counselors to start peer-supervision groups when they relocate to places where they do not already exist (Hiller and Rosenfield 2000; Likhite 2000; Zahm, McCarthy Veach, and LeRoy 2008).

PERSONAL EXPERIENCES

Genetic counselors may have personal experience with loss or illness. Not surprisingly, these experiences often breed interest in entering a helping profession. At times trainees are drawn to genetic counseling because they perceive that they can do it better than professionals who helped them or their family. Other times they admire the care they received and find themselves wanting to give back to others in similar ways. In either case, these past experiences can lead to interactions with clients that originate from one's own experience rather than from the clients' needs. These experiences can be assets to counselors, but only with the maturity and insight to differentiate responses to clients that may be more about oneself than the clients. This type of self-knowledge is very hard to achieve given that much of it happens subconsciously. Counselors who participate in peer supervision may share transcripts of their sessions where they suspect that their interactions with a client may reflect less-well-recognized aspects of their own needs or experiences. This may also be accomplished in professional supervision or psychotherapy.

Work in therapy can help us to differentiate when our personal experiences provide a benefit to empathic and cognitive understanding of clients from when they are a detriment or a self-focused detour. When counselors are working through their experiences in clinical work, it can often be a hindrance to achieving client-centered counseling. Processing personal losses and motivations to becoming a counseler is important to turning those experiences into professional assets. Seeking professional and peer help with issues of countertransference is professionally responsible and likely to elevate one's expertise in caring for clients.

Having personal experiences that provide insights into our clients' experiences in no way implies that one must have had experience with a genetic condition or personal loss to practice effectively. The majority of counselors have not had such experiences, but a disproportionate number have and benefit from insight into the relationship it has to one's work with clients. Learning to understand ourselves in our professional work as genetic counselors separately from our self-identity formed through our personal experiences is critical to establishing boundaries in our work. Over time a healthy integration of professional self and personal self should result in professionalism that allows personal experiences to inform our work.

COUNSELING EXPERIENCES

Our experiences with clients play a significant role in establishing our expectations of how current and future clients are likely to engage in genetic counseling. While counselors may perceive this as developing expertise in predicting how clients will respond to genetic information or testing options, another perspective is that counselors may be more likely to fall into routines based on their expectations of how new clients will respond and risk falling short in establishing therapeutic relationships and tailoring information delivery. Our past experiences lead to an ease in conveying genetic information, and it is understandable how that can result in an ill-considered practice routine that may limit efforts to learn the particularities of each client and his or her needs. Tailoring sessions to client priorities has been shown to lead to enhanced patient outcomes without taking more time (Eijzenga et al. 2014). The tendency to generalize clients' experiences to others is hard to resist and may largely be subconscious. It is common and an example where professional supervision can be an asset in helping all of us as counselors retain our ability to see each client as unique. We have never met the person and, thus, he or she is a stranger to us. This does not imply that counselors do not improve their insight and abilities to anticipate common client reactions with experience—quite the contrary. Instead, it suggests that the skills to assess client experiences, knowledge, preferences, and needs are of prime importance. We need to resist becoming complacent simply because our expertise with the genetics information is honed.

There is a paucity of literature that conveys the ways that genetic counselors grow personally from their professional work. The rewards lie in developing insights into the human condition, appreciating that people can emerge from suffering with renewed strengths, recognizing the power of short-term therapeutic relationships in providing opportunities for clients to help themselves, learning to accept that difficult things happen to good people, learning to give up some personal control, recognizing parents' abilities to manage enormous heartache, and bearing witness to effort, openness, willingness, and strengths that counselors can help clients find within themselves. Genetic counselors are gifted professionals who grow in their work, find new strengths, and are privileged to participate briefly in people's lives at challenging times. This is some of the most rewarding professional work when one pays focused attention to each client and his or her narrative and what it reveals about his or her experiences and needs.

SUMMARY

Counselors' traits, values, and beliefs find them well suited to provide highly skilled counseling. The biases and experiences that threaten these assets need to be kept at bay, and the responsibility lies with each of us to ensure that we are self-aware and have third parties, such as peers or a professional in a supervision group, to keep us continuing to learn about ourselves and our work so that we present our best selves when we engage with our clients.

REFERENCES

Ariely, D. 2009. *Predictably Irrational: The Hidden Forces That Shape Our Decisions.* New York: Harper.

Ash, E. 2017. "Motivational Interviewing in the Reciprocal Engagement Model of Genetic Counseling: A Method Overview and Case Illustration." *Journal of Genetic Counseling* 26: 300–11. https://doi.org/10.1007/s10897-016-0053-8.

Benoit, L. G., Patricia McCarthy Veach, and Bonnie LeRoy. 2007. "When You Care Enough to Do Your Very Best: Genetic Counselor Experiences of Compassion Fatigue." *Journal of Genetic Counseling* 16: 299–312. https://doi.org/10.1007/s10897-006-9072-1.

Buchanan, A. H., S. K. Datta, C. S. Skinner, G. P. Hollowell, and H. F. Beresford. 2015. "Randomized Trial of Telegenetics vs. In-Person Cancer Genetic Counseling: Cost, Patient Satisfaction and Attendance." *Journal of Genetic Counseling* 24: 961–70. https://doi.org/10.1007/s10897-015-9836-6.

Chen, A., P. M. Veach, C. Schoonveld, and H. Zierhut. 2017. "Seekers, Finders, Settlers, and Stumblers: Identifying the Career Paths of Males in the Genetic Counseling Profession." *Journal of Genetic Counseling* 25: 948–62. https://doi.org/10.1007/s10897-017-0071-1.

Cowan, Nelson. 2010. "The Magical Mystery Four." *Current Directions in Psychological Science* 19, no. 1: 51–57. https://doi.org/10.1177/0963721409359277.

Eijzenga, W., N. K. Aaronson, D. E. Hahn, G. N. Sidharta, and L. E. van der Kolk. 2014. "Effect of Routine Assessment of Specific Psychosocial Problems on Personalized Communication, Counselors' Awareness, and Distress Levels in Cancer Genetic Counseling Practice: A Randomized Controlled Trial." *Journal of Clinical Oncology* 20: 2998–3004. https://doi.org/10.1200/JCO.2014.55.4576.

Ellington, Lee, Bonnie J. Baty, Jamie McDonald, Vickie Venne, Adrian Musters, Debra Roter, William Dudley, and Robert T. Croyle. 2006. "Exploring Genetic Counseling Communication Patterns: The Role of Teaching and Counseling Approaches." *Journal of Genetic Counseling* 15, no. 3: 179–89. https://doi.org/10.1007/s10897-005-9011-6.

Ellington, Lee, Kimberly M. Kelly, Maija Reblin, Seth Latimer, and Debra Roter. 2011. "Communication in Genetic Counseling: Cognitive and Emotional Processing." *Health Communication.* 27, no. 7: 667–75. https://doi.org/10.1080/10410236.2011.561921.

Fagerlin, A., B. J. Zikmund-Fisher, and P. A. Ubel. 2011. "Helping Patients Decide: Ten Steps to Better Risk Communication." *Journal National Cancer Institute* 103: 1436–43. https://doi.org/10.1093/jnci/djr318.

Farrelly, Ellyn, Mildred K. Cho, Lori Erby, Debra Roter, Anabel Stenzel, and Kelly Ormond. 2012. "Genetic Counseling for Prenatal Testing: Where Is the Discussion about Disability?" *Journal of Genetic Counseling* 21, no. 6: 814–24. https://doi.org/10.1007/s10897-012-9484-z.

Ferrer, R. A., W. M. Klein, and K. A. Graff. 2017. "Self-Affirmation Increases Defensiveness toward Health Risk Information among Those Experiencing Negative Emotions: Results from Two National Samples." *Health Psychology* 36: 380–91. https://doi.org/10.1037/hea0000460.

French, David, E. Cameron, and J. S. Benton. 2017. "Can Communicating Personalised Disease Risk Promote Healthy Behaviour Change? A Systematic Review of Systematic Reviews." *Annals of Behavioral Medicine* 51: 718–29. https://doi.org/10.1007/s12160-017-9895-z.

Geller, G., E. S. Tambor, and G. A. Chase. 1993. "Incorporation of Genetics in Primary Care Practice: Will Physicians Do the Counseling and Will They Be Directive?" *Archives of Family Medicine* 2, no. 11: 1119–25.

Gervais, K. 1993. "Objectivity, Value Neutrality, and Nondirectiveness in Genetic Counseling." In *Prescribing Our Future: Ethical Challenges in Genetic Counseling*, edited by Dianne M. Bartels, Bonnie S. LeRoy, and Arthur Caplan, 119–30. New York: Aldine De Gruyte.

Han, Paul K., W.M. Klein, and N.K. Arora. 2011."Varieties of Uncertainty in Health Care: A Conceptual Taxonomy. *Medical Decision Making* 31, no. 6: 828–838.

Hiller, E., and J. M. Rosenfield. 2000. "The Experience of Leader-Led Peer Supervision: Genetic Counselors' Perspectives." *Journal of Genetic Counseling* 9: 399–410. https://doi.org/10.1023/A:1009402231506.

Hyatt, Jillian. 2012. "Countertransference in the Genetic Counseling Setting: One Counselor's Personal Journey." *Journal of Genetic Counseling* 21: 197–98. https://doi.org/10.1007/s10897-011-9435-0.

Injeyan, M. C., C. Shuman, A. Shugar, D. Chitayat, E. Atenafu, and A. Kaiser. 2011. "Personality Traits Associated with Genetic Counselor Compassion Fatigue: The Roles of Dispositional Optimism and Locus of Control." *Journal of Genetic Counseling* 20: 526–40. https://doi.org/10.1007/s10897-011-9379-4.

Joseph, Galen, Robin Lee, Rena J. Pasick, Claudia Guerra, Dean Schillinger, and Sara Rubin. 2019. "Effective Communication in the Era of Precision Medicine: A Pilot Intervention with Low Health Literacy Patients to Improve Genetic Counseling Communication." *European Journal of Medical Genetics* 62, no. 5: 357–367. https://doi.org/10.1016/j.ejmg.2018.12.004.

Joseph, G., R. J. Pasick, D. Schillinger, J. Luce, C. Guerra, J. K. Y. Cheng. 2017. "Information Mismatch: Cancer Risk Counseling with Diverse Underserved Patients." *Journal of Genetic Counseling* 26, no.5: 1090–1104. doi:10.1007/s10897-017-0089-4.

Kessler, Seymour. 1992. "Psychological Aspects of Genetic Counseling. VIII. Suffering and Countertransference." *Journal of Genetic Counseling*. https://doi.org/10.1007/BF00962826.

Kessler, Seymour. 1999. "Psychological Aspects of Genetic Counseling: XIII. Empathy and Decency." *Journal of Genetic Counseling*, no. 6: 333–43. https://doi.org/10.1023/A:1022967208933.

Likhite, Marisa Ladoulis. 2000. "The Interface between Countertransference and Projective Identification in a Case Presented to Peer Supervision." *Journal of Genetic Counseling* 9: 417–24. https://doi.org/10.1023/A:1009406332414.

Madeo, Anne C., Barbara B. Biesecker, Campbell Brasington, Lori H. Erby, and Kathryn F. Peters. 2011. "The Relationship between the Genetic Counseling Profession and the Disability Community: A Commentary." *American Journal of Medical Genetics Part A* 155, no. 8: 1777–85. https://doi.org/10.1002/ajmg.a.34054.

McAllister, M., and A. Dearing. 2015. "Patient-Reported Outcomes and Patient Empowerment in Clinical Genetics Services." *Clinical Genetics* 88, no. 2: 114–21. https://doi.org/10.1111/cge.12520.

McAllister, M., K. Payne, R. Mcleod, S. Nicholls, D. Dian, and L. Davies. 2008. "Patient Empowerment in Clinical Genetics Services." *Journal of Health Psychology* 13, no. 7: 895–905. https://doi.org/10.1177/1359105308095063.

Miller, Mary A., and Pamella Rae Stoeckel. 2017. *Client Education: Theory and Practice*. 3rd ed. Burlington, MA: Jones & Bartlett Learning.

National Society of Genetic Counselors. n.d. "NSCG Position Statement: Reproductive Freedom." Accessed March 12, 2019. https://www.nsgc.org/p/bl/et/blogid=47&ym=201006.

Nieuwhof, K., E. Birnie, and M. P. van den Berg. 2017. "Follow-up Care by a Genetic Counsellor for Relatives at Risk for Cardiomyopathies Is Cost-Saving and Well-Appreciated: A Randomised Comparison." *European Journal of Human Genetics* 25: 169–75. https://doi.org/10.1038/ejhg.2016.155.

Otten, E., E. Birnie, A. V. Ranchor, and J. P. Van Tintelen. 2015. "A Group Approach to Genetic Counselling of Cardiomyopathy Patients: Satisfaction and Psychological Outcomes Sufficient for Further Implementation." *European Journal of Human Genetics* 23: 1462–67. https://doi.org/10.1038/ejhg.2015.10.

Reeder, R., Patricia McCarthy Veach, Ian M. MacFarlane, and Bonnie S. LeRoy. 2017. "Characterizing Clinical Genetic Counselors' Countertransference Experiences: An Exploratory Study." *Journal of Genetic Counseling* 26: 934–47. https://doi.org/10.1007/s10897-016-0063-6.

Rentmeester, C. A. 2001. "Value Neutrality in Genetic Counseling: An Unattained Ideal." *Mental Health Care Philosophy* 4: 47–51.

Resta, Robert, Barbara Bowles Biesecker, Robin L. Bennett, Sandra Blum, Susan Estabrooks Hahn, Michelle N. Strecker, and Janet L. Williams. 2006. "A New Definition of Genetic Counseling: National Society of Genetic Counselors' Task Force Report." *Journal of Genetic Counseling* 15, no. 2: 77–83. https://doi.org/10.1007/s10897-005-9014-3.

Roter, D., L. Ellington, L. Hamby Erby, S. Larson, and W. Dudley. 2006. "The Genetic Counseling Video Project (GCVP): Models of Practice." *American Journal of Medical Genetics, Part C: Seminars in Medical Genetics* 142, no. 4: 209–20. https://doi.org/10.1002/ajmg.c.30094.

Sahhar, M., M. Bogwitz, E. Brown, R. Forbes, J. Greenberg, L. Hossack, and M. Menezes. 2008. "Letter to the Editor, *Journal of Genetic Counseling*: When You Care Enough to Do Your Very Best: Genetic Counselor Experiences of Compassion Fatigue." *Journal of Genetic Counseling* 17, no. 1: 139–40. https://doi.org/10.1007/s10897-007-9122-3.

Silver, J., C. Caleshu, S. Casson-Parkin, and K. Ormond. 2018. "Mindfulness among Genetic Counselors Is Associated with Increased Empathy and Work Engagement and Decreased Burnout and Compassion Fatigue." *Journal of Genetic Counseling* 27: 1175–1186. https://doi.org/10.1007/s10897-018-0236-6.

Ubel, Peter A., Karen A. Scherr, and Angela Fagerlin. 2018. "Autonomy: What's Shared Decision Making Have to Do with It?" *American Journal of Bioethics* 18, no. 2: W11–W12. https://doi.org/10.1080/15265161.2017.1409844.

Udipi, S., Patricia McCarthy Veach, and Bonnie LeRoy. 2008. "The Psychic Costs of Empathic Engagement: Personal and Demographic Predictors of Genetic Counselor Compassion Fatigue." *Journal of Genetic Counseling* 17: 459–71. https://doi.org/10.1007/s10897-008-9162-3.

Werner-Lin, A., J. L. McCoyd, and B. Bernhardt. 2016. "Balancing Genetics (Science) and Counseling (Art) in Prenatal Chromosomal Microarray Testing." *Journal of Genetic Counseling* 25: 855–67. https://doi.org/10.1007/s10897-016-9966-5.

Zahm, K. W., Patricia McCarthy Veach, and Bonnie LeRoy. 2008. "An Investigation of Genetic Counselor Experiences in Peer Group Supervision." *Journal of Genetic Counseling* 17: 220–33. https://doi.org/10.1007/s10897-007-9115-2.

CHAPTER 6

Applying Ethical Theories to Genetic Counseling Practice

INTRODUCTION

Ethical dilemmas are inherent to genetic counseling practice. Some examples of ethically challenging clinical scenarios encountered in genetic counseling might include clients who are reluctant to share critical genetic information with family members, patients who request testing that the counselor might think is inappropriate, misattributed paternity serendipitously discovered, exome sequencing that reveals a clinically important pathogenic variant unrelated to the primary reason for the testing, or monozygotic twins where one twin requests a genetic test for a dominant condition such as Huntington disease but the other twin does not want to know the information. You will undoubtedly encounter many other ethical dilemmas in your clinical practice. Clarke and Pettersson (2018) provide an excellent review of common ethical dilemmas in genetic counseling.

The social and cultural impact of genetic testing and counseling can create ethical divides. People with disabilities, their families, and their supporters may criticize prenatal screening as a form of modern-day eugenics, or, at the very least, as creating discrimination against people with disabilities. Poor or minority populations may have limited access to genomic medicine. Genetic testing may result in excessive costs, cause clinical harm, or be utilized when its benefits to the patient are unclear.

Ethical dilemmas are not always satisfactorily resolved. Nonetheless, they are an inevitable part of genetic counseling and learning to manage them is critical to your professional development.

This chapter is divided into three sections. The first section provides some basic background about bioethics. The second section discusses some of the more common frameworks of ethical analysis. The third section demonstrates a means to critically evaluate arguments for alternative resolutions for moral dilemmas and to use this evaluation to come to more thoughtful resolution of ethical dilemmas in genetic counseling practice.

BASICS

Bioethics applies philosophical frameworks for thinking about rightness and wrongness to research and practice in medicine and the life sciences. The term *bioethics* was coined in 1970 by Van Rensselaer Potter from the University of Wisconsin to describe "a discipline [that] would . . . help humankind toward rational but cautious participation in the processes of biological and cultural evolution" (Reich 1993, S7). The issues that arise in the practice of clinical genetics and genetic counseling have been central to bioethics since its inception.

The Importance of Humility

Genetic counseling professionals and their clients come from a variety of backgrounds and subscribe to a wide array of values and moral beliefs. It is unlikely that genetic counselors and clients will consistently share the same beliefs and values. However, even counselors and clients who have very different cultural backgrounds, life experiences, and outlooks on political and social questions can still find broad areas of ethical agreement.

Genetic counselors should approach their deliberations about ethics with humility and recognize limitations in their knowledge and life experience. Their cultural or family circumstances, rather than objective truths, will partly ground their personal or professional codes. Genetic counselors should be mindful of the basis of the ethical precepts of their practice and to be willing to evaluate points of conflict with clients and colleagues. For some, clinical supervision can be a mechanism to explore personal ethical conflicts and the implications they have for clinical practice (see Chapter 5). In other situations, consulting informally with colleagues or more formally with an institutional or professional ethics committee may help the counselor to resolve an ethical problem.

Approaching ethical dilemmas with humility also allows genetic counselors to learn from the diversity of perspectives that peers and clients bring to genetic counseling. The challenge of working with persons with different belief systems can result in counselors' deeper resolve in previously held ethics. For other counselors the challenges can lead to restructuring or reframing personal and professional values and beliefs. In either case, ethical discussions serve to improve genetic counselors' ethical understanding of their practice and improve the quality of their relationships with their clients, their colleagues, and society. Such humility is particularly critical when working with minorities, women, people with disabilities, and other people whose lack of power has resulted in their voices not being heard and suffering harm as a result.

Another reason for approaching ethical decision making with humility is that the current consensus about what is considered ethical may eventually become outdated. For example, for decades, the criteria for screening for genetic conditions were based on the Wilson–Jungner criteria (Wilson and Jungner 1968), which are based mostly on technical issues such as disease severity, disease prevalence, availability of effective interventions, and accurate testing. However, these criteria were delineated by clinicians, not by parents, who may have different priorities and perspectives than clinicians. In the twenty-first century, expanded newborn screening was justified on grounds of clinical utility since it could end the "diagnostic odyssey"—the process of making a genetic diagnosis in a patient that could sometimes last years—even in the absence of specific medical benefits from the diagnosis. Personal and parental utility is now given as much weight as clinical utility when deciding which conditions to include in newborn screening programs or exome and genome sequencing.

Another historical example of changing ethical values can be seen in the history of eugenics in the opening decades of the twentieth century. At the time, eugenics was not uncommonly viewed as a progressive philosophy that benefited society (Paul 1984). But after World War II and the atrocities committed in Nazi Germany, eugenics came to be identified as an unethical, racist practice; today the word is often used as an epithet or a criticism, particularly in discussions of prenatal diagnosis.

ETHICAL DECISION-MAKING FRAMEWORKS

The theoretical bases for bioethical deliberations have been evolving for centuries. Although some argue that there is no need for abstract theory in the discipline of bioethics, theory can provide the grounding necessary to enhance careful decision making in ethically difficult situations.

Western ethical theories continue to play critical roles in illuminating the conflicting values motivating ethical dilemmas as well as providing guidance in decision making. These theories of ethics seek to identify a defining characteristic that is present in all right actions and absent from all wrong actions.

Here we briefly describe some of the common frameworks employed in the consideration of bioethical dilemmas. Readers interested in a more in-depth discussion of these and other philosophies are directed to the Stanford Encyclopedia of Philosophy (http://plato.stanford.edu/contents.html).

Each ethical theory or perspective has strengths and weaknesses, and no one theory provides a universal construct for analyzing all biomedical dilemmas. Consequently, genetic counselors are cautioned against giving one philosophy or framework special status or weight in ethical conflicts in genetic counseling. Rather, counselors should view each perspective as providing "important but partial contributions to a comprehensive, although necessarily fragmented, moral vision" (Arras and Steinbock 1999, 9).

Describing the philosophical underpinnings of ethical paradigms can make for dense and difficult reading. To help relate the abstract to the concrete world of genetic counseling, keep the following theoretical scenario in mind as you read about different ethical approaches:

A fellow genetic counselor mentions to Noelle, a genetic counselor, that she seems confused and agitated. Noelle replies:

I just met with Antonia, woman who wants her healthy and normally developing fourteen-year-old daughter to have carrier testing for a familial BRCA mutation. Antonia, who has not had breast cancer, has a strong family history of breast cancer and a pathogenic BRCA1 mutation was identified first in her sister and, eventually, in Antonia. She told me that she wanted to test her teen daughter because she "wanted to make sure her daughter was aware of her cancer risks." When I brought up the option of testing when the daughter is older and could take an active role in the decision making, Antonia exploded with indignation and anger. She told me that it was her "right as a parent" to have her daughter tested. I told Antonia that we usually do not recommend testing children when there is no direct medical benefit to them. Antonia told me she understood that I had to follow the procedure but reiterated that she is adamant about carrier testing for her daughter.

I know that genetic testing of children can be beneficial for some children and their families, but it does not seem like the right thing to do in this case.

Noelle is faced with an ethical dilemma (of course, this cases also raises counseling issues about how to best address the mother's response, but put those aside for the moment). On the one hand, Noelle appreciates that parents generally have the authority and wisdom to make medical decisions for their children (Hanson and Thomson 2000) and they generally seek to enhance the well-being of their children. Moreover, she recognizes that preventing parents from exercising authority over their children runs the risk of damaging genetic counselors' relationships with their clients who are parent. On the other hand, Noelle believes the primary goal of genetic testing should be to enhance the *immediate* well-being of the child (American Society of Human Genetics and American College of Medical Genetics 1995), not to fulfill a parental request that is possibly grounded in the parent's personal psychological needs. She also believes that child's interest in genetic testing should be weighed when making decisions about offering testing to minors. Given the important issues outlined both for and against genetic testing, it is unclear if Noelle should facilitate genetic testing for Antonia's daughter.

The references by Shkedi-Rafid et al. (2015), Mand et al. (2012), and particularly McConkie-Rosell and Spiridigliozzi (2004) are helpful background reading in understanding the ethical complexities surrounding genetic testing of children for adult-onset conditions.

COMMON ETHICAL FRAMEWORKS

Deontology

The primary premises of deontology are (a) rightness and wrongness are located in one's motivations for acting rather than the actions themselves and (b) actions are wrong if they are motivated by anything other than one's recognition that one is morally obligated to do them. For example, an individual who bases her deliberation on religious commandments is appealing to a deontological framework, as is an individual who believes that our shared humanity obligates us to help others in need.

When applying deontology to clinical practice, a genetic counselor's tasks are (1) to define the moral duties relevant to the case and (2) to make a decision that best fulfills these moral obligations. Although seemingly simple, completing these two tasks can be challenging, particularly when there are conflicting moral duties.

Deontology focuses on motivations for actions rather than their consequences. Thus, an action with positive consequences would be ethically wrong if it were motivated by something other than recognition of a duty. Returning to Noelle's dilemma, imagine if Noelle falsely told the parent that BRCA testing is inaccurate in children, and the parent withdrew her request to have her daughter tested. Although Noelle may have achieved what she believed to be an ethical outcome, she has violated her duty to provide truthful and accurate genetic counseling.

Because deontology is concerned with motivations rather than consequences, it is difficult to hold individuals responsible for the consequences of their actions, even in cases in which we would intuitively assign blame. For instance, deontological theories cannot account for the intuition that revealing the whereabouts of a victim of domestic violence to her estranged spouse is morally wrong even though it conforms to duties to tell the truth.

Parker and Lucassen (2018) apply deontological analysis to the duty of confidentiality in a situation where a patient is reluctant to share with relatives information that is important for their medical care and treatment. The authors argue that because a familial factor led to the diagnosis of the condition in the patient, the counselor has a duty to inform other family members of the patient's clinical information. They further state that this policy should be shared upfront with the patient at the time of counseling, but it does not require the patient's consent. What do you think of their assessment?

Utilitarian Theories

In contrast to deontologists, utilitarians believe that an action's consequences determine its rightness or wrongness and that rightness or wrongness is quantifiable. In particular, utilitarians hold that actions are morally right in proportion to the number of individuals who will benefit from them and the degree to which those individuals benefit. For instance, a utilitarian might argue for a tax on large inheritances on the grounds that increased revenue for government programs allows a large number of people to receive important services and deprives heirs of relatively little.

According to utilitarian principles, when confronted with an ethical dilemma, a genetic counselor's tasks are to (1) survey alternative courses of action and their consequences and (2) choose the alternative that is most likely to bring about the greatest degree of positive consequences for the greatest number of people.

A utilitarian approach to Noelle's dilemma would be to consider the consequences of both facilitating testing and not facilitating testing and choosing the option that would promote the greatest good. Because there is no medical benefit to testing the fourteen-year-old daughter, and because it may interfere with the daughter's autonomy and freedom to make independent choices, one possible utilitarian resolution would be to not facilitate testing the daughter.

Genetic counselors often consciously or subconsciously use utilitarian ideas. This is not surprising, as the strengths of the utilitarian theories are that (1) they are based on rational deliberation of the consequences of actions and (2) they attempt to achieve the most benevolent outcome for a given dilemma. Moreover, utilitarian theories appeal to a genetic counselor's sense that particulars of situations can play important roles in the outcome of decision making.

Virtue Ethics

The group of moral theories considered under the umbrella of virtue ethics are specifically concerned with the role of character in moral decision making. The roots of these theories may be found in Plato and Aristotle in Greece and Confucius in China.

The general premise of virtue ethics is that the rightness or wrongness of an action is located in the habits of thought and affective dispositions (i.e., the character) that motivated it. For example, it would be wrong for Noelle to agree to test Antonia's daughter out of a need to be liked by her client or to avoid complaints rather than out of regard for her clients' well-being.

Although theories of virtue ethics are concerned with lifelong dispositions to think, feel, and act, they do not aim at codifying universal rules of action or decision making the way that deontological and utilitarian theories do. Instead, they seek to explain how having the right habits of thought and affective dispositions can allow individuals to identify and act on the ethically salient details of a situation.

In some cases the various habits of thought and affective dispositions (i.e., virtues) that ought to guide deliberation may conflict. In Noelle's situation, it could be argued that the virtue of friendliness is in direct conflict with the virtue of courage. The negotiation of conflicts within a theory may be found when applying virtually all ethical approaches to complicated genetic counseling dilemmas (Arras and Steinbock 1999), and counselors should remain critical when applying any ethical paradigm to professional dilemmas.

Several authors have applied virtue ethics to genetic counseling practice. For example, a study in which focus groups of geneticists and interviews with patients were conducted to look at the informed consent process in clinical genetic testing found that despite the best efforts of clinicians, many patients came away from the consent process with a poor understanding of the provided information (Samuel et al. 2017). The authors concluded that information-based consenting does not meet patient needs. Instead, they proposed that consent should be based on ethical values of honesty, openness, and trustworthiness.

Feminist Ethics

Feminist ethics attempts to revise, reformulate, or rethink those aspects of traditional Western ethics that "depreciate or devalue women's moral experience" (Tong 2008, 1), as well as the experiences of other traditionally disadvantaged groups (such as the disabled and persons of color). Feminist philosophy positively revalues characteristics such as caring, emotionality, intuitiveness, and partiality that other theories of ethics may treat as negative or irrelevant to ethical decision making.

Historically, feminist ethics is particularly relevant to the genetic counseling profession. The National Society of Genetic Counselors (NSGC) working group that formulated the original NSGC Code of Ethics published in 1992 specifically developed the code with feminist ethics in mind (Judith Bendkendorf, personal communication).

Some feminist ethicists have criticized prenatal diagnosis (e.g., Browne 2017; Dickenson 2016), arguing that it results in commodification and commercialization of pregnancy and that it is not gender neutral. Unlike many other ethical perspectives, feminist ethicists may also analyze prenatal diagnosis from a justice and power perspective. Some feminist ethicists have also argued that prenatal diagnosis devalues the rights of disabled people and the non-disabled women who often are responsible for raising disabled children (Parens and Asch 2000; Patterson and Satz 2002). On the other hand, some disability rights activists have criticized feminists for not supporting people with disabilities when feminists support prenatal diagnosis and abortion as primarily a matter of women's reproductive choice.

Hesse-Biber (2014) uses a feminist approach to explore the process by which women who are BRCA positive socially construct and understand their risk status and the management strategies they chosoe to follow, and in a later study (Hesse-Biber and An 2017) examined the medical decisions made by male BRCA mutation carriers.

Returning to Noelle's dilemma, a feminist analysis might examine how the internal and societal expectations that shape Antonia's role as a woman and mother might inform her decision to request testing for her daughter. The focus shifts then to her rights and responsibilities as a woman and mother to allow her to make the best possible decision for herself and her daughter, based on caring and emotionality.

Casuistry

According to casuistry, deliberators appeal to similarities with other cases rather than general ethical principles to ground their decisions. Casuistry may be likened to the process used to develop case law (Beauchamp and Walters 1999) where judges evaluate legal cases and make authoritative judgments that serve as the bases for judgments in subsequent cases with similar features. For instance, if she took this approach, Noelle would base her decision whether to test Antonia's daughter on her response to past encounters with demanding clients instead of considerations about obligation, character, or maximizing benefits to mother and daughter.

One of the advantages of using a case-based approach is that genetic counselors are not bound by the requirements of impartiality and responding to similar cases in exactly the same way. Rather, they are free to use their skills in discernment to identify important similarities in cases, to evaluate alternative paths to resolution, and to make use of practical judgment.

Principilism

In their influential book *The Principles of Bioethics* (originally published in 1977) Tom Beauchamp and James Childress (1994) assert that bioethical decision making need not conform to a single theory of ethics. Rather, it should make use of principles common to a variety of systems of ethics. This approach has become widely used both in clinical practice and in the formation of health care and research policy. For example, *The Belmont Report: Ethical Principles and Guidelines for the Protection of Human Subjects of Research*, an influential document on human subjects research, uses principilism as its backbone (National Commission 1979). In principilism, four basic ethical principles—autonomy, nonmaleficence, beneficence, and justice—are considered when faced with an ethical dilemma, but no single principle takes priority over the others.

Autonomy is the right to self-governance. In other words, it allows for liberty of action, self-determination, privacy, respect for persons, and individuality. Three conditions are essential for autonomy: (1) liberty (independence from external influences), (2) agency (capacity to act), and (3) competence (the ability to perform a task).

Let's return to Noelle's situation. If Noelle understands autonomy as freedom from external compulsion, she may believe that she ought to exclusively focus the counseling on the medical information related to BRCA testing rather using the session to discuss the relationship between Antonia's values and goals and BRCA testing. However, if she understood autonomy as the right to be determined by one's own values and aims, Noelle, Antonia, and her daughter would discuss their beliefs about BRCA testing and the goals and values that motivated Antonia to seek it. Noelle might also introduce issues that other clients have deliberated when making decisions regarding BRCA testing, which the teen and her mother may not have considered. In this case, Noelle's aim would be to enhance the teen's decision making by challenging her to consider multiple perspectives, some of which may be vastly different from her own. To mitigate the risk of manipulation and coercion, the counselor would explicitly address these issues in the genetic counseling session.

Nonmaleficence is the obligation not to harm another. The principle of nonmaleficence is related to the principle of beneficence (see next section). In the context of genetic counseling, concerns about maleficence generally center not on physical harms but rather on psychological or social harms. For example, carrier screening may be conducted with nominal physical harm (i.e., pain associated with the blood draw) for those who elect to have screening done. However, screening does have a significant potential for causing psychological and social harm. For instance, due to misinformation and misunderstanding of correct information offered by sickle cell screening programs, many clients were unnecessarily stigmatized and discriminated against. Some insurance companies charged higher rates or denied coverage to African Americans with sickle cell trait (Hudson et al. 1995) (though this would not currently be legal, under the Genetic Information Nondiscrimination Act of 2008).

The principle of nonmaleficence also plays a prominent role in dilemmas involving research protocols. For example, the genetic counselor, as part of the research team, is obligated by the principle of nonmaleficence to ensure that enrollment in the protocol does not lead the client to experience unnecessary harm. This duty can be particularly complicated to meet when the physical and/or psychological and social risks and benefits of a given protocol are that which the researchers seek to understand. For example, a number of genetic counseling research studies of exome/genome sequencing have sought to understand the psychological and social effects of learning about risks for conditions that were unrelated to the primary reason for testing to begin with. Concerns have been raised that clinical susceptibility testing might have a significant negative impact on clients' psychological well-being and adherence to health behaviors such as screening regimens.

Beneficence is the moral obligation to contribute to the welfare of other individuals rather than merely refraining from doing harm to them. Beneficence requires that the genetic counselor and client be in a relationship and that the counselor be a "trustee" of the client's welfare (Schmerler 1998); this is often called a fiduciary relationship. The specific obligations based on beneficence depend on the type and degree of relationship between individuals. For example, if a woman requests information and counseling about Fragile X syndrome as part of a genetic counseling appointment, a genetic counselor is obligated to meet the client's request in light of established counseling guidelines (McIntosh et al. 2000). However, if a fellow cocktail party guest asks for information about Fragile X syndrome, the counselor may only be obligated to encourage the guest to view the National Fragile X Foundation website and to speak to her own health care provider regarding her concerns. In the first case the counselor has a professional relationship with the client. In the second case, the counselor has a much less binding relationship with the individual requesting assistance. Thus, the nature of the relationship between a genetic counselor and individuals seeking the counselor's expertise has a bearing on the counselor's moral obligation and responses to counseling requests.

In light of beneficence, genetic counselors ought to facilitate genetic testing options that have the highest efficacy and safety and should caution clients from utilizing questionable testing practices and medical procedures, as well as making decisions based on the outcomes of these practices and procedures. Beneficence also supports encouraging clients to get involved in support groups and genetic disease networks.

Justice requires that a genetic counselor's behavior remains consistent and that the counselor act fairly with clients and other professionals. In the simplest sense, "Like cases should be treated alike." Differences in the counselor's behavior between two cases should be justified by appealing to relevant differences in the cases.

As noted in Noelle's situation, BRCA testing may not be in the immediate best medical interests of the daughter because that information would not be used to guide the daughter's medical care for at least a decade, and testing could potentially violate her autonomy. But with other genetic disorders, testing the daughter could be medically and ethically justified. If, for instance, the disorder in question was familial adenomatous polyposis due to an APC gene mutation, then the detection of the mutation in the daughter would lead to a critical change in her health care—that is, she would need to undergo colonoscopy to assess her polyp burden and to determine if she has an asymptomatic cancer.

When using principilism, a genetic counselor must consider each principle in relation to the given dilemma. The strength and weight of arguments based on each principle will vary. It is the process of articulating arguments in light of each principle, weighing them, and balancing and counterbalancing them that help resolve the dilemma. In practice, a genetic counselor may decide that arguments in support of Alternative A are founded on one set of principles, whereas arguments in support of Alternative B are based on another set. In other situations, arguments based on the same principle may actually support two diametrically opposed alternatives!

In a qualitative study of a large Lynch syndrome kindred, Lorraine Cowley (2016) examined the moral reasoning behind patients' decisions to undergo—or not—genetic testing. Participants typically framed the decision to undergo testing as "common sense"—not as a choice but rather as a moral imperative. The choice of testing was simultaneously viewed by patients as both an autonomous choice and a responsibility. Test accepters defended the right of any relative "not to know" while simultaneously acknowledging the importance of testing.

CASE DELIBERATION

In the previous sections, we discussed the philosophical traditions genetic counselors have drawn on when deliberating professional ethical dilemmas. In this section, we present practical steps for wrestling with dilemmas and deciding on courses of action.

Is It Really a Dilemma?

Given the nature of genetic counseling practice, it is common for genetic counseling cases to include a variety of ethical issues. By definition, dilemmas arise when the reasons for opposing actions or judgments *seem at first glance to be equally good* (or equally bad). Noelle's case is a clear example of an ethical dilemma because it is unclear if the counselor should facilitate BRCA testing in the daughter.

Not all ethical *issues* generate bona fide ethical *dilemmas*. That is, in some cases ethical issues are raised but the course of action to address them is straightforward. For example, a client was referred to a prenatal genetic counselor for teratogen counseling. At the onset of the appointment, the client explained that she had told her husband that she was concerned about the effects of alcohol on her pregnancy (she had been "partying heavily" for a few days around the time of conception). In truth, the client was primarily worried about the fact that the father of the baby was likely not her husband, but rather a man of African descent (the client was of Scandinavian descent). She wanted to have prenatal paternity testing but could not locate the man she suspected was the father. Moreover, she didn't want to tell her husband about her infidelity, so his blood could not be used for paternity testing either. She told the counselor that she feels that her only choice is to tell her husband that *the counselor said* that there is a significant risk to the fetus due to the alcohol exposure and then to have an abortion. The client also asked the counselor to write a follow-up letter, which she plans to show her husband, emphasizing the teratogenic effects of the alcohol.

As a professional, the counselor is obligated to help clients adapt to difficult information, make decisions, and enhance relationships. She accepts that clients can interpret the same information in many ways and that some may use their interpretations to promote unethical endeavors. However, the client has requested that the counselor abet the client's decision to lie to her husband by writing a skewed follow-up letter. If the counselor were to write such a letter, she would be working against her own values of integrity and competence. Such a letter also would not promote truth and trust in the couple's relationship and would be in direct conflict with the traditions and practices of other health professionals. Thus, although this case illustrates an important ethical issue, counselors' responsibilities toward clients, it does not pose a genuine dilemma. It is clear that ethically and legally, the counselor may only write a letter that actually reflects the information presented in the case. She is not at liberty to alter these facts in order to abet a client's lie.

Clarification of Facts

In other apparent ethical dilemmas, clarifying the facts can expedite resolution. Although this is a seemingly self-evident point, it deserves note. For example, a genetic counselor met with a thirty-five-year-old man with colon cancer, along with his three siblings who came along for support. During the session, the genetic counselor discussed the potential implications of genetic test results for the patient and his siblings and promised to work with the siblings if the testing indicated that the patient had a hereditary cancer syndrome.

Two weeks later the test results showed that the patient had Lynch syndrome. When the counselor again raised the issue of implications for his siblings, he replied that would never tell his siblings because it was too difficult, and he didn't want them to worry about their own cancer risks if any of them were to prove to have Lynch syndrome. As the client was late for an appointment with his oncologist, the client would not engage the counselor in further discussion about the meaning of her comment. The next day the counselor contacted the client by telephone to probe further regarding his comment. The client stated that that he was just expressing his fears and anxieties about his siblings' developing cancer, but that he fully intended to inform them once he completed his chemotherapy in a few months. Right now, he was so physically worn down that he did not have the emotional wherewithal to discuss Lynch syndrome testing with his family.

In other cases, clarifying facts does not make the appropriate course of action any more evident. In these cases, further deliberation is needed. For example, if in the preceding case the patient was insistent about not informing his relatives about their risks for Lynch syndrome, the counselor would be in the difficult position of balancing respect for the patient's privacy against the immediate and serious medical implications for his siblings whom she promised to work with.

General Steps for Case Analysis

Other texts (Maley 1994; Schmerler 1998) offer detailed descriptions of the steps a genetic counselor should take when deliberating an ethical dilemma in the genetic counseling context. The general steps of case analysis are listed in Box 6.1. In the first step, the genetic counselor uses her assessment and information-gathering skills. The counselor goes beyond just clarifying the facts to assessing the relationship of these facts to each of the parties involved in the conflict. In the second step, the counselor seeks to enumerate the ethical conflicts and evaluate resources that would be helpful in evaluating these conflicts. Resources may include discussions of moral philosophies, professional codes of ethics, and institutional policy documents. Consultation with colleagues and the NSGC Ethics Subcommittee or another professional ethics committee can be invaluable at this step. Likewise, consultation with professional ethics committee members may be very helpful with the third step: weighing the alternatives and making a decision. However, beyond making the decision, the third step requires that the factors for implementing the decision be laid out and evaluated. Finally, in the fourth step the genetic counselor assesses the decision-making and implementation process in light of its ultimate outcome. This enables the

> *Box 6.1*
> **STEPS FOR CASE ANALYSIS**
>
> <u>Assess the situation</u>: Who is involved? What happened? What stakes does each party have in the outcome of this case?
> <u>Identify the ethical problems and considerations:</u> What are the problems? How have other cases been resolved? What resources are needed to help find resolution for this dilemma?
> <u>Make a decision:</u> What are the arguments (and their weights) for each alternative decision? What ethical constructs support the decisions? Who will ultimately decide? Who will implement the decision?
> <u>Evaluate the decision after implementation:</u> How did the decision work out in the short run? In the long run? How can this problem be avoided in the future?
>
> *Adapted from Maley (1994) and Schmerler (1998).*

counselor, as well as other colleagues, to make the most out of the work done in the prior three steps. In some cases, the fourth step will culminate in the development of a new written policy or formal clarification of an established policy.

The case analysis process is useful because it causes genetic counselors to account for and evaluate the arguments in a systematic and thoughtful way. This decreases the likelihood that important information and critical arguments will be overlooked. However, not all arguments supporting a decision are equally strong. That is, although a reason may be given to support a given alternative, when carefully considered the argument may be found to be irrelevant or weak, at best, and thus less worthy of consideration. So, how can genetic counselors better present and evaluate the arguments that are brought forward in a discussion of an ethical dilemma?

CRITERIA FOR EVALUATING ETHICAL ARGUMENTS

Here we build on the discussion on the process of case analysis by providing a complementary means to present and evaluate ethical arguments concerning genetic counseling dilemmas. This method is based on that described and evaluated by Beabeu (1995). According to this method, an argument may be evaluated on the four major criteria listed in Box 6.2. Often consideration of one criterion will lead to further thinking regarding another. This is expected and welcomed in this deliberative process.

> **Box 6.2**
> **CRITERIA FOR EVALUATING ARGUMENTS**
>
> 1. Adequate description of the points of conflict
> 2. Consideration of all interested parties
> 3. Adequate analysis of probable consequences of alternative decisions for all interested parties
> 4. Evaluation of the obligations of those involved in the dilemma
>
> *Adapted from Bebeau (1995).*

Description of the Points of Conflict

When making a thoughtful argument regarding a dilemma, it is not enough to just "name" an issue germane to the case (e.g., autonomy). Rather, a genetic counselor must work to describe the nature of the conflict. Analogous to data gathered through qualitative means, description enables the nuances of conflicts to shine through. Furthermore, describing the outstanding points of conflict often leads to the illumination of the less apparent, but no less problematic, points. For example, Box 6.3 lists the points of conflict in the previously described case, assuming that the client told the genetic counselor that he would not share his Lynch syndrome results with his siblings. An argument for (or against) having the genetic counselor support this client's request requires a response to each of these conflicts.

> **Box 6.3**
> **POINTS OF CONFLICT IN LYNCH SYNDROME EXAMPLE**
>
> - Client's right to privacy versus siblings' right to information that is critical to their health, especially after it had been discussed during the initial genetic counseling session
> - Individual rights (individual's DNA) versus family rights (does the whole family own its DNA?)
> - Legal limitations on sharing patient data (Health Insurance Portability and Accountability Act of 1996 [HIPAA]) versus ethical duty to warn siblings of health risks

> *Box 6.4*
> **INTERESTED PARTIES IN LYNCH SYNDROME CASE**
>
> PATIENT
> Right to privacy of genetic information
> Fragile emotional status during chemotherapy and grappling with his mortality
> Right to protect the psychological health of his siblings
>
> SIBLINGS
> Established relationship with the genetic counselor because they were present during the counseling session in which the sharing of test results had been addressed
> Right to information that can reduce their risk of developing cancer if testing shows they do have Lynch syndrome
> Right to avoid high-risk screening and risk-reducing surgery if testing shows they do not have Lynch syndrome
>
> GENETIC COUNSELOR
> Right to have her own moral code respected
> Right to practice genetic counseling
> Interest in abiding by her professional ethical code
> Interest in maintaining a good reputation as a genetic counselor
> Interest in fostering a therapeutic genetic counseling relationship with her client and his family
> Interest in making sure siblings are advised of appropriate screening and risk-reducing strategies
>
> SOCIETY
> Interest in promoting health of citizens
> Interest in appropriate utilization of health resources
> Interest in avoiding harm to citizens (e.g., avoiding unnecessary surgeries, reducing the risk of cancer, detecting cancers at earlier stages)

Consideration of All Interested Parties

As in many genetic counseling situations, individuals other than the client may have a vested interest in the ultimate action taken in a given dilemma. When considering all those who have a stake in the decision, it is important to consider the rights and interests not only of individuals but also groups, such as families, organizations, and society at large. Box 6.4 lists the considerations of those with stakes in the case of the client who planned to withhold his Lynch syndrome genetic results from his family.

Analysis of Consequences

Once the genetic counselor has considered the points of conflict and the interested parties in the dilemma, attention should turn to analyzing the consequences of given alternatives. A strong argument does not require listing and evaluating *every* possible consequence. Rather, a valid argument requires consideration of "those [outcomes] that have a good probability of occurring or those that would have very serious consequences even if the probability of occurrence is not particularly high" (Bebeau 1995, 17). Likewise, it is important to keep in mind that the impact an action may have on a given person or organization in the short run may seem minor, but the effects in the long run may seem more grave. Box 6.5 lists several possible consequences to the genetic counselor in the hypothetical case. Box 6.6 a complete argument for (or against) the genetic counselor's decision must adequately consider the consequences of this decision on the other interested parties (listed in Box 6.4) as well.

Study of the Obligations of Those Involved

Finally, the genetic counselor must evaluate the obligations of those involved in the case to each other. The major tenet of the ethic of care (that decision making takes place in the context of relationships) directly supports this criterion. A genetic counselor should enumerate both the obligations and, more importantly, the reasons behind each of the obligations evaluated in terms of values, principles, and character (Bebeau 1995). Box 6.5 lists some of the genetic counselor's obligations and their justifications in the case of the man withholding Lynch syndrome results from his family. The obligations of the other interested parties (listed in Box 6.4) should also be considered for a thorough argument.

We believe that by combining the case analysis process outlined in Box 6.1 with the criteria for a strong argument outlined in Box 6.2, a genetic counselor may make thoughtful decisions based on sound moral reflection. With that said, genetic counselors must keep in mind that human nature dictates that everyone is fallible, and so even using a cogitative approach

> *Box 6.5*
> **CONSEQUENCES FOR THE COUNSELOR IN THE LYNCH SYNDROME CASE**
>
> If the genetic counselor elects to support the client's request to not share test results with siblings:
>
> - She will maintain her established relationship with her client.
> - She may feel content because she supported her client's right to privacy.
> - She may feel her actions helped her avoid legal vulnerability.
>
> Alternatively...
>
> - She may feel significant remorse for putting the siblings at greater health risk if they do not know their cancer risks and appropriate management strategies.
> - She may suffer harm to her reputation. That is, others may view the counselor as amoral or immoral.
>
> If the counselor elects NOT to support the client's request to not share test results with family:
>
> - She will lose her established relationship with her client.
> - She may feel remorse for not being able to meet her client's needs.
> - Others may view her as paternalistic, or perhaps as inappropriately intruding into family dynamics.
> - It is possible that the patient was right, and his siblings develop serious psychological sequelae from knowing their risk status
>
> Alternatively...
> - She may feel content that she did not participate in an act that could have resulted in significant harm to the siblings.

cannot safeguard anyone completely from error. For some counselors, and in some situations, such a structured approach is neither feasible nor worthwhile. We expect, however, that generally using a deliberative approach with professional dilemmas will enable a genetic counselor to be better equipped to analyze current and future professional dilemmas and find resolutions that better meet the needs of their clients, colleagues, society, and themselves (Box 6.6).

> Box 6.6
> ### OBLIGATIONS OF THE GENETIC COUNSELOR IN THE LYNCH SYNDROME CASE
>
> - <u>To conduct herself with integrity:</u> As a person and a health care professional, the genetic counselor is required to be truthful. Honesty is essential for healthy personal and professional relationships.
> - <u>To treat her client with respect:</u> As a therapeutic genetic counselor, the counselor seeks to understand and support her client. Without respect, these other goals of the genetic counseling relationship cannot be attained.
> - <u>To enhance the relationship between the client and his family:</u> After the counseling session, the client will likely return to his usual relationship and interactions with his siblings. It is the client who must live with the ultimate ramifications of not sharing the test results with his family. The genetic counselor is obligated to help the client negotiate with his siblings his decision to not share his genetic test results.
> - <u>To seek clarification of the rules/regulations of the medical center regarding this issue and abide by those:</u> As an employee of the cancer center, it is the genetic counselor's responsibility to be aware and follow the rules and regulations of her employer. Generally, rules and regulations were put in place after careful thought and consideration of the needs of clients and employees. They are there to support employees, not hinder practice.
> - <u>To seek counsel from a professional ethics committee:</u> This dilemma has many facets. Although it is important for the genetic counselor to be part of the decision making, it is also vital that harms are minimized to both her and the other parties involved. This may be better achieved through the involvement of the ethics committee.
> - <u>To promote the health of the clients' siblings</u>
> - <u>To promote the betterment of citizens in the United States:</u> Women have fought in the United States to be seen as equal in moral and social status to men. The genetic counselor must work to ensure that the female position (particularly in the microcosm of the family) is upheld.

REFERENCES

American Society of Human Genetics & American College of Medical Genetics. 1995. "Points to Consider: Ethical, Legal, and Psychosocial Implications of Genetic Testing in Children and Adolescents." *American Journal of Human Genetics* 57, no. 5: 1233–41.

Arras J, Steinbock B. 1999. *Ethical Issues in Modern Medicine*. Mayfield Publishing Company, California City, CA.

Beauchamp, T. L., and J. F. Childress. 1994. *Principles of Biomedical Ethics*. 4th ed. New York: Oxford University Press.

Beauchamp, T. L., and L. Walters. 1999. "Introduction to Ethics." In *Contemporary Issues in Bioethics*, edited by T. L. Beauchamp and L. Walters, 5th ed., 1–32. Belmont, CA: Wadsworth Publishing Company.

Bebeau, M. J. 1995. *Moral Reasoning in Scientific Research*. Bloomington: Indiana University Press.

Browne, T. K. 2017. "Why Parents Should Not Be Told the Sex of Their Fetus." *Journal of Medical Ethics* 43: 5–10. doi:10.1136/medethics-2015-102989.

Clarke, A., and C. Wallgren-Pettersson. 2018. "Ethics in Genetic Counseling." *Journal of Community Genetics* 10, no. 1: 3–33. doi.org/10.1007/s12687-018-0371-7.

Cowley, L. 2016. "What Can We Learn from Patients' Ethical Thinking about the Right 'Not to Know' in Genomics?" *Bioethics* 30: 628–35.

Dickenson, D. 2016. "Feminist Perspectives on Human Genetics and Reproductive Technologies." *Encyclopedia of Life Sciences* (Wiley OnLine). doi:org/10.1002/9780470015902.a0005592.pub3.

Hanson, J. W., and E. J. Thomson. 2000. "Genetic Testing in Children: Ethical and Social Points to Consider." *Pediatric Annals* 29(5): 285–91.

Hesse-Biber, S. 2014. "The Genetic Testing Experience of BRCA-Positive Women: Deciding between Surveillance and Strategy." *Qualitative Health Research* 24: 773–89.

Hesse-Biber, S., and C. An. 2017. "Within-Gender Differences in Medical Decision Making Among Male Carriers of the BRCA Genetic Mutation for Hereditary Breast Cancer." *American Journal of Men's Health* 11: 1444–59.

Hudson, K. L., K. H. Rothenberg, L. B. Andrews, M. J. Kahn, and F. S. Collins. 1995. "Genetic Discrimination and Health Insurance: An Urgent Need for Reform." *Science* 270, no. 5235: 391–93.

Maley, J. A. 1994. *An Ethics Case Book for Genetic Counselors*. Charlottesville: University of Virginia.

Mand, C., L. Gillam, M. B. Delatycki, and R. E. Duncan. 2012. "Predictive Genetic Testing in Minors for Late-Onset Conditions: A Chronological and Analytical Review of the Ethical Arguments." *Journal of Medical Ethics* 38: 519–24.

McConkie-Rosell, A., and G. A. Spiridigliozzi. 2004. "'Family Matters': A Conceptual Framework for Genetic Testing in Children." *Journal of Genetic Counseling* 13: 9–29.

McIntosh, N., L. W. Gane, A. McConkie-Rosell, and R. L. Bennett. 2000. "Genetic Counseling for Fragile X Syndrome: Recommendations of the National Society of Genetic Counselors." *Journal of Genetic Counseling* 9, no. 4: 303–25.

National Commission for the Protection of Human Subjects of Biomedical and Behavioral Research. 1979. *The Belmont Report: Ethical Principles and Guidelines for the Protection of Human Subjects of Research*. Washington, DC: US Department of Health, Education, and Welfare.

Parens, E., and A. Asch, editors. 2000. *Prenatal Testing and Disability Rights*. Washington, DC: Georgetown University Press.

Parker, M., and A. Lucassen. 2018. "Using a Genetic Test Result in the Care of Family Members: How Does the Duty of Confidentiality Apply?" *European Journal of Human Genetics* 55: 285–86. doi:10.1038/s41431-018-0138-y.

Patterson, A., and M. Satz. 2002. "Genetic Counseling and the Disabled: Feminism Examines the Stance of Those Who Stand at the Gate." *Hypatia* 17: 118–42.

Paul, D. B. 1984. "Eugenics and the Left." *Journal of the History of Ideas* 45: 567–90.

Rapp, R. 2000. *Testing Women, Testing the Fetus: The Social Impact of Amniocentesis in America*. New York: Routledge.

Reich, W. T. 1993. "How Bioethics Got Its Name." *Hastings Center Report* 23, no. 6: S6–S7.

Schmerler, S. 1998. "Ethical and Legal Issues." In *A Guide to Genetic Counseling*, edited by D. L. Baker, J. Schuette, and W. Uhlman, 249–75. New York: Wiley-Liss.

Shkedi-Rafid, S., A. Fenwick, S. Dheense, and A. M. Lucassen. 2015. "Genetic Testing of Children for Adult-Onset Conditions: Opinions of the British Adult Population and Implications for Clinical Practice." *European Journal of Human Genetics* 23: 1281–85. doi:10.1038/ejhg.2014.221.

Tong, R. 2008. "Feminist Ethics." In Stanford Encyclopedia of Philosophy. https://plato.stanford.edu/entries/feminism-ethics/.

Wilson, J. M. G., and G. Jungner. 1968. *Principles and Practice of Screening for Disease*. Geneva: WHO. Available from: http://www.who.int/bulletin/ volumes/86/4/07-050112BP.pdf.

CHAPTER 7

Conflict of Interest and the Code of Ethics

In Chapter 6 we discussed ethical theories and how they might be applied to direct patient care. In this chapter we address the ethical issues that can arise in interactions with our colleagues and in genetic counselors' roles in the broader context of the delivery of health care services—specifically, conflicts of interest (COIs). We then look at two professional resources for guidance in making ethical choices in both the clinical and professional domains—the National Society of Genetic Counselor (NSGC)'s Code of Ethics and the NSGC's Ethics Advisory Group.

CONFLICT OF INTEREST

There are many ways to define COI, but the Institute of Medicine (2009)'s definition is commonly used: *a set of circumstances that creates a risk that professional judgment or actions regarding a primary interest (e.g., a patient's best interests) will be unduly influenced by a secondary interest (e.g., financial or professional gain for the counselor).*

COIs can occur in all areas of genetic counseling employment—clinics, academic centers, commercial laboratories, administration, and research. They can also occur in professional activities—developing practice guidelines, educational presentations, authorship, manuscript and grant review, and duties carried out as part of professional organizations such as the NSGC and the American Board of Genetic Counseling (ABGC).

The NSGC's Code of Ethics (http://www.nsgc.org/p/cm/ld/fid=12) contains several explicit statements regarding COIs (Section I, Items 5–7, and Section II, Item 2):

- Identify and adhere to institutional and professional conflict of interest guidelines and develop mechanisms for avoiding or managing real or perceived conflict of interest when it arises.
- Acknowledge and disclose to relevant parties the circumstances that may interfere with or influence professional judgment or objectivity or may otherwise result in a real or perceived conflict of interest.
- Assure that institutional or professional privilege is not used for personal gain.
- Clarify and define their professional role(s) and relationships with clients, disclose any real or perceived conflict of interest, and provide an accurate description of their services.

The NSGC also has published COI policies for organizational activities and duties. These policies apply to organizational staff and leaders; educational programs and publications; practice guidelines; exhibitor/sponsor rules; partnerships; name, logo, and trademark use; and website advertising (http://www.nsgc.org/p/cm/ld/fid=13).

The NSGC has developed a toolkit to educate genetic counselors about how to think about and manage COIs and to identify resources to help navigate the tricky waters of COIs (https://www.nsgc.org/p/cm/ld/fid=552%20http:/www.nsgc.org/page/gc-conflict-of-interest). In addition, most employers have COI guidelines and resources that employees are expected to abide by.

Forms of COI

COIs may entail financial and nonfinancial gain. The Institute of Medicine report (2009) suggests that there are five possible forms of COI, all of which may fall within the scope of the genetic counseling profession:

- <u>Tangible financial COI</u>—direct financial tie to the success of a product (e.g., salary or commission based on the sales of a genetic test). For example, the American College of Medical Genetics specifically recommends against testing polymorphisms in MTHFR, a gene that produces methylenetetrahydrofolate reductase, an enzyme involved in folic acid metabolism. Despite this recommendation, some

alternative-care providers offer MTHFR testing for many of their patients and then recommend provider-developed products for patients who are found to have polymorphisms that may alter folate levels, which are purported to affect the risk of a wide range of health conditions.
- Intangible financial COI—receiving payment for a service tied to the success of a product or research (e.g., a paid speech or editorial)
- Personal COI—personal beliefs or goals that are tied to research. For example, a genetic counselor who believes that a certain intervention is a particularly good way to provide genetic counseling to patients in crisis situations conducts a study that purports to show the effectiveness of the intervention. However, when the manuscript is sent for review, the reviewers identify flaws in research design and statistical analysis that undermine the counselor's conclusions. In this scenario, the COI created by the counselor's personal beliefs blinded her to the shortcomings of the research.
- Professional COI—if a genetic counselor gains professionally from the success of a study. For example, if the counselor in the above example about personal COI also stood to earn a promotion from an important publication or could have qualified for institutional funding to attend a meeting to present her study, then there would have been both personal and professional COIs.
- Institutional COI—interests of an institution or institutional official affect the design, reporting, review, or oversight of research (e.g., failing to reporting of adverse medical outcomes, suppressing research critical of institutional policies or practices). In 1999, Jesse Gelsinger, an eighteen-year-old patient with ornithine transcarbamylase deficiency, participated in a gene therapy trial at the University of Pennsylvania. Several days after his treatment, he died as a result of an immune response to the viral vector used to effect the gene transfer. It was later discovered that the lead researcher in the trial, a university employee, was a founder of the company that developed the technology used in the trial, and the university had financial interests in the company.

Commentators and researchers have tried to distinguish among actual COI (a real and tangible situation that clearly compromises judgment), perceived COI (such as when patients or the news media perceive a COI even though the counselor feels that one does not exist), and potential COI (professional judgment *could* be compromised). But these distinctions are not clear cut and are difficult to separate. A COI can exist even if no direct harm has occurred. In other words, a COI is usually real; the question becomes whether (1) it intentionally or unintentionally resulted in patients received less than standard of care or being physically or emotionally harmed, (2) it impaired the genetic counselor's judgment, or (3) the counselor received personal or professional gain.

Why Does COI Matter?

There is a tendency to think of COI in terms of large-scale financial scandals with profound and serious effects, and certainly these have occurred in the business sector. One example is the experience with Wells Fargo Bank (https://en.wikipedia.org/wiki/Wells_Fargo_account_fraud_scandal), where pressure to meet sales goals resulted in accusations that employees created millions of savings and checking accounts without the account holders' approvals. Of note, the bank had very clear and detailed policies on COI: "Team members must avoid conflicts of interest or the appearance of conflicts of interest in their personal and business activities. The appearance of a conflict of interest may be just as damaging to the reputation of Wells Fargo as the existence of an actual conflict of interest" (https://www.sec.gov/Archives/edgar/data/72971/000119312509127827/dex991.htm).

Another example of a large-scale conflict of interest in a company with a strong COI policy was the action by the Volkswagen Group to install software in millions of cars that could detect when a car's carbon monoxide emissions were being tested and then change the engine's output to meet those standards (Castille and Foltz 2018). Like Wells Fargo, Volkswagen has a very clear code of ethics with a COI policy: "Therefore, it is imperative that all situations from which conflicts of interest could arise be avoided" (https://www.volkswagenag.com/en/group/compliance-and-risk-management/compliance.htmlf).

Fortunately, large-scale COI scandals have not emerged in the genetic counseling profession to date. However, articles in the *New York Times* and the *Boston Globe* suggested that some genetic counseling patients perceived that their genetic counselors' undisclosed COI—being employed by a testing laboratory or receiving speaking fees from a laboratory—may have influenced their genetic counseling (Daley 2016; Pollack 2012). Whether or not the counselors' COI actually compromised the quality of the service they provided is, on one level, irrelevant. The problem is that a financial COI may have been present and may not have been properly disclosed to the patient, and some patients felt this compromised their care. The corrosive effects on public trust in genetic counselors could be devastating to the profession (Kelly 2016).

Thus, not only is it critical for the profession and employers to have clearly stated COI policies, but mechanisms must be in place to address instances of COI when they arise to determine their veracity, accuracy, and effects. Just as critical is a means for individual counselors to assess their own perception of the situation, ideally through professional supervision with a noninvolved third party (see the discussion later in the chapter about subconscious perceptions of COI).

KEY CONCEPTS IN UNDERSTANDING COI

To effectively address and manage financial COI for the clinical, laboratory, or research genetic counselor, it is helpful to understand some key concepts.

COI is often viewed as a conscious choice: that is, one makes a choice out of personal greed to knowingly engage in unethical behavior that results in financial enrichment of oneself and/or one's employer. Medical and nonmedical professions have a sometimes less-than-stellar track record of situations where professionals betrayed their fiduciary relationship for the sake of personal, professional, or employer gain. Clearly that possibility must be guarded against in the genetic counseling profession.

As noted, to date the genetic counseling profession has not been marked by scandals of greed, deception, or cheating. Thus, we can only provide theoretical examples of self-aware COI in the genetic counseling profession:

1. A clinical counselor has set up a high-risk cancer clinic. The economic justification for establishing the clinic that the counselor used to convince the hospital administration is that it would generate significant downstream revenue from increased utilization of imaging and surgical services. The counselor calculates how many additional breast magnetic resonance imaging scans would be required to cover the clinic's overhead. She then proceeds to falsify patients' breast cancer risk calculations such that a significant number of patients wind up with a lifetime breast cancer risk of 20% or greater, the risk cutoff at which breast MRI screening is recommended.
2. A research counselor is part of a large grant-funded study looking at the value of exome sequencing of low-birth weight infants in the neonatal intensive care unit. Worried that enrollment is too low and that the grant will not be renewed, with the result that the counselor would lose his job, he lowers the newborn weights on the enrollment forms so that a greater number of newborns are now apparently eligible for the study.
3. A lab-employed counselor has the role of encouraging obstetrical offices to do their own hereditary cancer testing, without referral to a genetic counselor. After providing a brief training session to the office staff at a busy obstetrics practice, she realizes that the staff really does not

understand the implications or appropriate usage of hereditary cancer testing. However, she is concerned that she will not meet her (perhaps unstated) quota for new accounts. She therefore tells the staff and her employer the practice is ready to initiate a hereditary cancer testing program.

All readers would agree that the genetic counselors made unethical and perhaps illegal choices in the above scenarios. But thinking about COI as only a conscious process is a very narrow and not altogether accurate understanding of how COIs arise and operate. There is now a considerable body of psychological research that strongly suggests that a more accurate way of thinking about COI is that it is primarily an *unconscious* process tied into the very nature of the human brain, the underlying motivations of human behavior, and how we perceive and justify our own actions.

The concept of subconscious COI is based on studies that indicate that most decisions and choices are made on such a deeply subconscious level that we are usually never aware of the underlying psychological processes. Our choices are typically based on personal gain. Without knowing it, on a subliminal level, individuals can make decisions without intending to be unethical or even consider that their behavior has ethical implications, even though observers would regard the decisions as unethical. The unconscious mind "tampers and rearranges self-knowledge so as to ensure that a certain view is maintained but retains no conscious belief that such tampering has taken place" (Chugh et al. 2005, p. 8). In other words, we all have blind spots that do not allow us to see our choices or behavior as unethical or inappropriate.

This has been shown to be equally true for people who firmly believe themselves to be highly ethical and who are in professions where they believe they are making decisions that are always in the best interests of their clients. *In other words, COI is the norm for human behavior and is the result of normal psychological processes.*

It can be remarkably easy to justify ethical transgressions, especially about matters that do not have serious adverse outcomes. For example, think of an office coffee fund to which everyone is supposed to contribute. Those who don't contribute to the fund because they are not regular coffee drinkers may still feel justified in helping themselves to a cup of coffee every now and then because "I'm not *really* a coffee drinker so I don't feel obliged to contribute to the coffee fund; besides, I *deserve* a free cup of coffee because I clean the office kitchen every now and then even though I don't make a mess in there." At heart, one knows that this behavior is not quite ethical, and hence the need to justify it to oneself by pointing out other selfless behaviors conducted on behalf of the office.

This is a harsh view of human nature but one that is amply supported by psychological research and case studies (Bazerman et al. 2006; Bertrand, Chugh, and Mullainathan 2005; Chugh, Bazerman, and Banaji 2005; Eldred 2015; Feldman, Gauthier, and Schuler 2013; Gino, Moore, and Bazerman 2009; Greenwald 1980; Haidt and Joseph 2004; Moore et al. 2006; Moore, Tanlu, and Bazerman 2010; Morar and Washington 2016; Paharia et al. 2009; Sah and Fugh-Berman 2013; Seligman 2002; Shu, Gino, and Bazerman 2011; Tenbrunsel et al. 2012).

This model is similar to a large body of literature on our inherent and unacknowledged biases toward persons of other races, age, body type, sexuality, disability, religion, etc. While many of us may believe that we are open-minded and embrace human diversity, at a deeply subconscious level we have biases that guide our behaviors to a far greater degree than we would be comfortable acknowledging or are even capable of acknowledging.

Thus, perhaps a more constructive way of viewing COI is that it is part of the professional growth and development of the genetic counselor. COI is not a transgression committed by a few undisciplined and greedy individuals. It is a natural result of human psychology and the at times conflicting interests that might arise when we have both our own interests and patients' interests to watch out for. As such, it requires regular education, self-reflection, and ideally professional supervision, much in the way that countertransference is a professional issue that is a normal occurrence rather than a pathological deviation. Of course, a critical distinction is that countertransference is essentially unavoidable whereas counselors can take some measures to reduce COI.

While COI guidelines are critical, alone they are insufficient to curb the potential effects of COI (see the Wells Fargo and Volkswagen examples cited earlier in the chapter). In fact, some studies have suggested that having guidelines may paradoxically and subtly encourage inappropriate behaviors. Some people who have undergone COI training and education can come to believe that because of the training they received, they certainly would have the expertise to identify any of their own actions and behaviors as being unethical or inappropriate. COI training can itself result in a blind spot in which one convinces oneself of a personal awareness about COI that may be misleading.

This paradigm can help explain how financial and other scandals develop. Individuals subconsciously make small unethical choices, but the conscious mind interprets them as perfectly ethical. Not uncommonly, ethical transgressions can spread virally—that is, if coworkers notice the ethical transgression, they tend to use this observation to justify their own similar transgressions: "Well, John does and so does Mary, so why shouldn't I? If it were so wrong, others wouldn't be doing it!" Such contagion of unethical behavior can become even more virulent when the transgressor is a supervisor or company executive. In these situations, those involved likely made a small series of unethical choices that their subconscious minds had convinced them were entirely appropriate and ethical, until one day the situation crossed the threshold into a full-fledged scandal. This phenomenon has been observed in many of the large corporate scandals of the last twenty-five years. Tenbrunsel et al. (2012) described this phenomenon as *ethical fading*—"the process by which, consciously or subconsciously, the moral colors of an ethical decision fade into bleached hues that are void of moral implications. Self-deception allows for the ethical discoloration of a decision, or the fading away of its ethical aspects." (p. 4)

A related concept is called "motivated blindness," the tendency to overlook the unethical behaviors of others when they are in our best interests. Examples of motivated blindness could be a hospital ignoring the unethical or inappropriate behavior of a surgeon who is a significant revenue source for the hospital, or administrators overlooking the inappropriate ethics and practices of a researcher who is very successful at securing large research grants. Motivated blindness can also be directed internally (i.e., the inability to see the negative consequences of our own actions and choices that we benefit from).

To suggest that genetic counselors are not subject to unconscious COI would be to say that the profession is unique among all of humanity. Genetic counselors are not unethical; rather, it is extraordinarily difficult to act ethically, more difficult than we can know. Paradoxically, the more ethical we claim to be, the more difficult it may be to see our own ethical shortcomings.

A common response to COI accusations is to say that personal or employer gain was the furthest thing from their minds, and accusing us of such behavior is highly inaccurate and inappropriate; we were entirely motivated by the best interests of our client. Counselors may point to professional codes of ethics, which typically include strong moral statements against COI, suggesting somehow that the mere existence of guidelines invalidates such charges.

THE PERCEPTION OF COI

The perception that a COI exists arises when an outsider—a patient, a reporter, a colleague—thinks that a genetic counselor has acted unethically because the counselor has a financial tie to an entity, either direct (salary, commission, stock options, etc.) or indirect (speaking fees, consulting fees, meals, gifts, etc.) and those ties resulted in recommendations or behaviors that were not primarily in a patient's best interests. In such situations, because of unconscious COI, it is difficult for individual counselors to determine on their own if they actually engaged in unethical behavior. There are, of course, multiple sides to every story and all of them are only partially true, even though each party may firmly believe that their version is the truth.

The above-mentioned newspaper articles can be viewed as examples of the perception of COI. These articles are warning shots across our bow, trying to alert us to the potential damage that can be done to the profession if there is the perception of COI, whether or not it actually resulted in substandard counseling practices. The articles may frustrate and anger us, but, really, we should be thankful for them. They are trying to wake us up from our ethical slumber.

On one level, it does not matter if the COI accusations in these articles are accurate. What matters is that patients—the life blood of the genetic counseling profession—may become hesitant to utilize our services if they think that those services will be influenced, consciously or not, by counselors' financial affiliations and employer demands. We need to be proactive about COI to reduce the chances that such articles will appear, or at least have adequate resources in place to show that the profession has taken very serious steps to reduce the possibility of COI influencing patient care. We may even have to acknowledge that sometimes our critics have a point.

Genetic counselors may face many situations during the course of their careers that could result in COI. Below are some examples of situations that could be viewed as creating COIs. We are not implying that genetic counselors in these situations are necessarily engaging in unethical practices. Rather, we are trying to encourage you to apply what you have read in this chapter to increase your personal and professional awareness and understanding of the complicated topic of COI.

- A hospital-based genetic counselor in a breast cancer clinic is required by his employer to refer patients for imaging studies only to a specific radiology group affiliated with the hospital, even if another radiology group not affiliated with the hospital utilizes imaging technology that provides better screening and diagnostic services than the hospital-based group can provide.
- A hospital-based genetic counselor refers patients at high risk of developing ovarian cancer to a specific gynecologic oncologist in a group practice because the counselor has a close and rewarding professional relationship with the oncologist, even though all the oncologists in the group are equally competent. The counselor does not benefit financially

from this practice, but the oncologist does, to the detriment of the income of the oncologist's partners.
- A hospital-based genetic counselor is funded by a commercial laboratory to give a paid talk at an expensive restaurant about the general benefits of exome sequencing, after which laboratory employees deliver a sales pitch for their exome-sequencing test.
- A commercial laboratory employs genetic counselors in a private hospital to provide genetic counseling for patients who may use the laboratory's test products, although the counselors are not required to use the laboratory exclusively.
- At national conferences, after-hours parties and events are sponsored by commercial entities that offer products and services that counselors may utilize in their clinical practices.
- Commercial entities offer small, low-cost gifts to counselors, such as pens, coffee mugs, and tote bags.
- A laboratory provides free pre-test genetic counseling to patients who use the laboratory's genetic tests.
- A laboratory provides free post-test genetic counseling to patients who use the laboratory's genetic tests.
- A research genetic counselor conducts research on potential non–alcohol-related behavioral problems in babies born with fetal alcohol syndrome that is funded by a national lobbying and support organization representing the interests of the wine and spirits industry.

In summary, managing COI is important for maintaining public trust and confidence, as well as professional integrity. COIs typically occur at a subconscious level and are often unavoidable, regardless of the employment setting of a genetic counselor. Like countertransference, it can be very difficult to identify and acknowledge when COI may have affected one's clinical judgment; professional supervision may be needed in some situations.

PROFESSIONAL RESOURCES: NSGC CODE OF ETHICS AND ETHICS ADVISORY GROUP

A code of ethics is not an ethical theory. Rather, it is an attempt to utilize ethical theories to develop guidelines for professional and clinical practice. It sets specific moral expectations for members of those societies, and to that extent they invoke virtue ethics (Lo 1995). The code is a statement of beliefs about the responsibilities and conduct of members of a particular profession and often set its standard of behavior. Although a given professional dilemma can be resolved using common sense and appealing to one's personal or institutional moral code, a professional society's code of ethics can be especially helpful in situations in which these resources do not readily delineate a course of action.

Codes of ethics may be written in language that makes them seem legally binding. However, in general there is little a society's membership may do in order to ensure that its members abide by the established code of ethics (Beauchamp and Walters 1999). Regardless, "[b]y adopting a code of ethics, a professional organization demonstrates to society (the public) that it accepts responsibility for defining professional conduct, for sensitizing its members to important ethical issues, and for affirming professional accountability" (Benkendorf et al. 1992, 32).

The code of ethics was initially adopted in 1992 and revised in 2006. In January 2017, the NSGC adopted the most recent version of the Code of Ethics (http://www.nsgc.org/p/cm/ld/fid=12). The NSGC Code of Ethics Review Task Force has recommended that the Code of Ethics be reviewed every five years to determine if it needs to be updated (Senter et al., 2018).

The Association of Genetics Nurses and Counsellors (http://www.agnc.org.uk/about-us/agnc-documents/code-of-ethics/), the Canadian Association of Genetic Counsellors (https://www.cagc-accg.ca/doc/code%20of%20ethics%20e-070628.pdf), India's Board of Genetic Counseling (http://www.geneticcounselingboardindia.com/uploads/3/4/8/5/34857846/bgc_code_of_ethics___sop.pdf), and the Australasian Society of Genetic Counsellors (https://www.hgsa.org.au/documents/item/22), among others, have codes of ethics very similar to the NSGC's.

To emphasize the importance of ethical behavior among genetic counselors, the Membership Committee of the NSGC requires new members to indicate that they will abide by the Code of Ethics (National Society of Genetic Counselors Annual Report, 1999). The ethics subcommittee of the NSGC utilizes the Code of Ethics when providing counsel to members struggling with professional dilemmas, as well as when evaluating NSGC policy documents.

The NSGC Code of Ethics is based on the ethic of care and the importance of four relationships:

- Genetic counselors themselves
- Genetic counselors and their clients
- Genetic counselors and their colleagues
- Genetic counselors and society

The NSGC Code of Ethics sets the *ideal* standard of ethical practice among genetic counselors. Likewise, it emphasizes education and professional development in response to ethical conflicts, in contrast to punitive measures for substandard behaviors (Benkendorf et al. 1994). This approach was taken in order to espouse a professional environment that fosters and enhances professional growth and development. Moreover, the Code of Ethics does not seek to specifically address all issues that a genetic counselor might face or give clear direction; rather, its intention is to provide a general framework for professional conduct. The NSGC Code of Ethics also draws on principilism (see Chapter 6), stating that it is based on principles such as veracity, objectivity, integrity, mutual respect, and client autonomy.

Sometimes it can be easier to use the Code of Ethics to judge the ethical behavior of others than it is to use it to assess your own behaviors and choices. Because genetic counselors strive to be ethical, we tend to view our own behaviors in a better light than others may view us. The NSGC's Ethics Advisory Group can offer guidance to members in evaluating and choosing courses of action for ethical dilemmas arising in clinical and professional practice. The Ethics Advisory Group is charged with doing the following:

- Interprets, reviews, and revises the NSGC Code of Ethics as it applies to the practice of individual members, as well as to the NSGC's relationship with its membership and society at large. This includes providing informal and formal ethics consults to NSGC members on request.
- Reviews NSGC documents to ensure that they are not in conflict with the NSGC Code of Ethics.
- Develops educational activities and materials on ethical issues pertinent to NSGC members.

The input of the Ethics Advisory Group can be particularly helpful for situations in which the ethical course of action might not be readily apparent to a genetic counselor caught in the midst of an ethically complicated situation.

REFERENCES

Bazerman, M. H., D. A. Moore, P. E. Tetlock, and L. Tanlu. 2006. "Reports of Solving the Conflicts of Interest in Auditing Are Highly Exaggerated." *Academy of Management Review* 31, no. 1: 1–7.

Beauchamp, T. L., and L. Walters. 1999. "Introduction to Ethics." In *Contemporary Issues in Bioethics*, 5th ed., 1–32. Belmont, CA: Wadsworth Publishing Company.

Benkendorf, J. L., N. P. Callanan, R. Grobstein, S. Schmerler, and K. T. FitzGerald. 1994. "Code of Ethics: Day-to-Day Applications." *Journal of Genetic Counseling* 3, no. 3: 245–61.

Benkendorf, J. L., N. P. Callanan, R. Grobstein, S. Schmerler, and K. T. FitzGerald. 1992. "An Explication of the National Society of Genetic Counselors (NSGC) Code of Ethics." *Journal of Genetic Counseling* 1, no. 1: 31–40.

Bertrand, M., D. Chugh, and S. Mullainathan. 2005. "Implicit Discrimination." *American Economic Review* 95, no. 2: 94–98.

Castille, C. M., and A. Fultz. 2018. "How Does Collaborative Cheating Emerge? A Case Study of the Volkswagen Emissions Scandal." Proceedings of the 51st Hawaii International Conference on System Sciences. https://scholarspace.manoa.hawaii.edu/bitstream/10125/49901/1/paper0014.pdf Accessed May 22, 2018.

Chugh, D., M. H. Bazerman, and M. R. Banaji. 2005. "Bounded Ethicality as a Psychological Barrier to Recognizing Conflicts of Interest." In *Conflicts of Interest*, edited by D. Moore, G. Loewenstein, D. Cain, and M. H. Bazerman, 74–95. London: Cambridge University Press.

Daley, B. 2016. "When Baby Is Due: Genetic Counselors Seen Downplaying False Alarms." *Boston Globe*, March 6, 2016, https://www.bostonglobe.com/metro/2016/03/05/when-baby-due-genetic-counselors-seen-downplaying-false-alarms/bBC0KAFVidJASkkOiMg6DI/story.html, accessed June 17, 2017.

Eldred, T. W. 2015. "The Psychology of Conflict of Interest in Criminal Trials." American Bar Association. http://www.americanbar.org/content/dam/aba/events/professional_responsibility/2015/May/Conference/Materials/psychology_of_conflicts_of_interest.authcheckdam.pdf, accessed June 18, 2017.

Feldman, Y., R. Gauthier, and T. Schuler. 2013. "Curbing Misconduct in the Pharmaceutical Industry: Insights from Behavioral Ethics and the Behavioral Approach to Law." *Journal of Law and Medical Ethics* 41, no. 3: 620–28. doi:10.1111/jlme.12071.

Gino, F., D. A. Moore, and M. H. Bazerman. 2009. "See No Evil: Why We Fail to Notice Unethical Behavior." In *Social Decision Making: Social Dilemmas, Social Values, and Ethical Judgments*, edited by R. M. Kramer, A. E. Tenbrunsel, and M. H. Bazerman, 241–63. New York: Psychology Press.

Haidt, J., and C. Joseph. 2004. "Intuitive Ethics: How Innately Prepared Intuitions Generate Culturally Variable Virtues." *Daedalus* 133: 55–67.

Institute of Medicine. 2009. *Conflict of Interest in Medical Research, Education, and Practice*. Washington, DC: National Academies Press. doi:10.17226/12598.

Kelly, T. 2016. "Conflicts about Conflict of Interest." *Cambridge Quarterly of Healthcare Ethics* 25, no. 3: 526–35. doi:10.1017/S0963180116000177.

Lo, B. 1005. *Resolving Ethical Dilemmas: A Guide for Clinicians*. Baltimore: Williams and Wilkins.

Moore, D. A., L. Tanlu, and M. H. Bazerman. 2010. "Conflict of Interest and the Intrusion of Bias." *Judgment and Decision Making* 5: 37–53.

Moore, D. A., P. Tetlock, L. Tanlu, and M. Bazerman. 2006. "Conflicts of Interest and the Case of Auditor Independence: Moral Seduction and Strategic Issue Cycling." *Academic Management Review* 31: 10–29. doi:10.5465/amr.2006.19379621.

Morar, N., and N. Washington. 2016. "Implicit Cognition and Gifts: How Does Social Psychology Help Us Think Differently about Medical Practice?" *Hastings Center Report* 46, no. 3: 33–43. doi:10.1002/hast.588.

Paharia, N., K. S. Kassam, J. D. Greene, and M. H. Bazerman. 2009. "Dirty Work, Clean Hands: The Moral Psychology of Indirect Agency." *Organizational Behavior and Human Decision Processes* 109, no. 2: 134–41. doi:10.1016/j.obhdp.2009.03.002.

Pollack, A. 2012. "Conflict Potential Seen in Genetic Counselors." *New York Times*, July 13, 2012, http://www.nytimes.com/2012/07/14/business/conflict-potential-seen-in-genetic-counselors-paid-by-testing-companies.html, accessed June 17, 2017.

Sah, S., and A. Fugh-Berman. 2013. "Physicians Under the Influence: Social Psychology and Industry Marketing Strategies." *Journal of Law and Medical Ethics* 41: 665–72. doi:10.1111/jlme.12076.

Seligman, J. 2002. "No One Can Serve Two Masters: Corporate and Securities Law after Enron." *Washington University Law Quarterly* 80, no. 2: 449–520.

Senter, L., R. L. Bennett, A. C. Madeo, S. Noblin, K. E. Ormond, K. W. Schneider, . . . A. Virani; National Society of Genetic Counselors Code of Ethics Task Force (COERTF). 2018. "National Society of Genetic Counselors Code of Ethics: Explication of 2017 Revisions." *Journal of Genetic Counseling* 27: 9–15. https://doi.org/10.1007/s10897-017-0165-9.

Shu, L., F. Gino, and M. H. Bazerman. 2011. "Dishonest Deed, Clear Conscience: When Cheating Leads to Moral Disengagement and Motivated Forgetting." *Personality and Social Psychology Bulletin* 37, no. 3: 330–49. doi:10.1177/0146167211398138.

Tenbrunsel, A. E., K. A. Diekmann, K. A. Wade-Benzoni, and M. H. Bazerman. 2012. *The Ethical Mirage: A Temporal Explanation as to Why We Aren't as Ethical as We Think We Are*. http://www.hbs.edu/faculty/Publication%20Files/08-012.pdf, accessed June 18, 2017.

CHAPTER 8

Relational Genetic Counseling

Testing and telling is not itself counseling, but where the essential process is the relationship, it is counseling.

(Patterson 1975, 12)

Genetic counseling goals resemble those of most health care encounters. To varying degrees, health care providers aim to effectively convey health information; recommend treatment or prevention activities; facilitate decision making; and promote effective coping with health risks or a medical condition. Genetic counseling addresses similar goals in the context of heritable risk or identification of a congenital anomaly, rare disease, or genetic condition. Clinical practice extends these goals to include psychological counseling to address cognitive and affective responses to inherited risks and related concerns. This chapter highlights the relational components of the counseling relationship that are essential to the success of these goals.

Genetic counseling can involve a one-time encounter (generally lasting thirty to ninety minutes), depending on the client's needs and the setting (https://www.nsgc.org/page/genetic-counselor-workforce-initiatives-532). There may be two counseling sessions when predictive testing is offered and results are subsequently returned, or multiple sessions over years when managing a child with a genetic condition, congenital anomaly, or developmental disorder. Within most service delivery models, genetic counselors have the opportunity to establish a therapeutic alliance with their clients to address the impact of the health threat of genetic information.

The Genetic Counseling Reciprocal Engagement Model (REM; Veach, Bartels, and LeRoy 2007) situates the relationship between the provider and patient at the center of practice. The REM conceptualizes the professional, clinical relationship as one that encompasses five tenets:

1. Genetic information is key.
2. The relationship is integral to genetic counseling.
3. Patient autonomy must be supported.
4. Patients are resilient.
5. Patients' emotions "make a difference."

Development of the model and its endorsement occurred within a meeting of twenty-three graduate program directors working together to address a recognized training need.

While the model represents a step forward for defining the profession, evidence from genetic counseling practice was not used to inform its development, nor has it been subsequently assessed. The REM, like other clinical practice models, falls short in conveying the means to establish the relationship and the skills needed to act within it. Thus, genetic counseling must turn to other sources to inform a practice model. One important source can be found in relational psychology, the core of clinical psychology theories (Patterson 1975). Relational psychology defines the elements of the clinical relationship that make it therapeutic for clients.

ESTABLISHING CLIENT SAFETY AND TRUST

For relational counseling to occur, the counselor needs to establish a safe environment for the client. In a trusting encounter, the client can come to feel cared about and valued, and these responses leave clients more open to sharing their thoughts and feelings. When counselors actively listen, clients come to trust that the provider is working to understand them and has their best interests in mind. These relational gains help lead to a working alliance.

The amount of effort undertaken by the counselor to establish a safe and trusting relationship should be realistic. That is, it should reflect the degree of threat posed by the genetic information or risk. Specifically, prenatal clients objectively face a small risk that their fetus is affected with a condition. This reality should be used to gauge the time spent and the depth of the relationship. Within a trusting relationship, clients need to be helped to make well-considered and informed decisions about prenatal screening. This includes exploration of their beliefs and values relevant to identification of a fetal abnormality. The art of relational counseling in the prenatal setting is in establishing a sufficient therapeutic alliance to prepare the minority of women and their partners who unknowingly carry an affected fetus for the challenging decisions ahead without frightening the majority who do not. When a fetus is found to be affected, the counseling is some of the most clinically challenging. As such, it is the counselor's objective to establish a sufficient alliance with the woman or couple that she or they will trust the counselor to help them through a very difficult decision. To accomplish this "sufficient" alliance, the counselor takes into account that the majority of clients are carrying a healthy fetus and will not face a difficult decision. As such, some preparation for an affected fetus is called for but should not reach the point where it burdens the majority for no good reason. Expert genetic counselors work to achieve this balance.

This general guidance fails to consider individual differences that arise when parents are particularly anxious or perceive themselves to be at high risk even if they are not. In these cases, more time is spent on understanding the client's needs and a stronger therapeutic alliance is needed. And for those patients referred after the risk to the fetus is determined to be high or a condition has been identified, it is more challenging to establish a therapeutic alliance as the couple is likely in a crisis. Although clients in crisis can be helped, the work occurs without a therapeutic alliance. See Chapter 9 for discussion of crisis counseling.

One of the arguments against making an effort to establish a therapeutic relationship in genetic counseling is time limitations, yet unquestionably a therapeutic alliance may be established in a single session. Evidence to support this claim comes from a randomized controlled trial in cancer genetics (Eijzenga et al. 2014). Prior to the session, patients were asked to indicate their priorities for discussion and their affective concerns. Following the trial's design, in half of the cases the genetic counselors reviewed the patient's checklist prior to the session. The sessions in each arm were of a similar length. Yet in the sessions where the counselors had reviewed the checklist prior, the issues of highest priority to clients were addressed by the counselor much earlier in the sessions. Further, patients were significantly more satisfied in the sessions where the checklist informed the case. These data suggest that client needs can be better met with an emphasis on client priorities early in sessions. Negotiating a session goal, setting expectations, and ensuring that client priorities are addressed promptly can lead to a therapeutic alliance.

Further, research in psychotherapy has found that positive client outcomes are frequently associated with higher expectations to receive help. This evidence suggests that assessing clients' receptivity to being helped is important to its success. Indeed, genetic counseling most often begins with a negotiation between counselor and patient about the most desirable outcomes. This is referred to as "contracting" in the National Society of Genetic Counselor (NSGC)'s practice guidelines. The objective is to generate an agreement between the professional and client about the goals for the session and the work needed to accomplish them. Most health care encounters do not overtly include contracting as the purpose of the visit is obvious or intuitive. For example, a person with back pain seeing an orthopedist presumes to learn more about the source of the back pain and remediation. Health care providers may begin their sessions by checking in on the purpose of the visit, but most often they do not engage in contracting.

In contrast, in genetic counseling, often in prenatal sessions, clients may be uncertain why they are seeing a counselor, or why their physician referred them (Bernhardt, Biesecker, and Mastromarino 2000). Starting a relationship unaware of its purpose makes it more difficult for clients to actively engage in negotiating or "contracting" about what will be accomplished. When clients have a reasonable idea of why they have been referred, such as to discuss genetic testing for inherited cancer risks to inform surgical decisions, the cancer genetics specialty service still may be sufficiently unfamiliar to them that their expectations are ill formed. For these reasons, genetic counseling includes contracting as a key practice competency to aid in establishing clients' expectations and to meet their explicated needs.

Contracting suggests an actively negotiated exchange where clients express their concerns and the counselor reinforces how genetic counseling may be of use in addressing them. Yet what should be such an exchange between counselor and client in the name of contracting often resembles a declaration by the genetic counselor. The counselor will state what will happen in the session and then asks if that is okay with the client. Specifically, the counselor may say, "First we will start by taking your family history, followed by a medical history. Then we will discuss genes and, if we make a diagnosis, how the condition is inherited. Does that sound alright to you?" Within a framework of relational counseling, alternative ways to begin sessions are preferable. Effective contracting engages the client and teaches the counselor about the unique needs of the client and family. When counselors declare an agenda, they do not mean to ignore the opportunity to get to know their client. Rather, it happens after we have repeated experiences with clients saying they are unsure what they will gain from the session and don't know what to expect, or the tendency for clients to recite the same need—for example, to arrive at a diagnosis for their child's condition. As a result, counselors reflexively present an agenda rather than invite clients to state their needs.

If clients are unsure what to expect from genetic counseling, counselors still can be effective in contracting by working with them to learn what they were thinking about the visit before they came or what they told others about why they were meeting with a genetic counselor. Almost all clients can answer these queries and advance their understanding about what is likely to occur in their session by engaging with the counselor. They can then add their hopes for what will occur in the session and the counselor can offer goals that may be achieved and a contract, of sorts, agreed upon.

ESTABLISHING THE RELATIONSHIP

The therapeutic relationship begins with a working alliance within an atmosphere of sincere interest and trust. Relationship counseling is the cornerstone of psychotherapeutic counseling (Patterson 1975). All types of psychotherapeutic counseling depend on the quality of the relationship established between counselor and client. Specific core conditions are common to effective counseling (Norcross and Wampold 2011). Given the central role of the relationship in the REM of genetic counseling, relational counseling can be appropriated for its evidence-based conditions that achieve positive client outcomes.

As presented thus far, a relational approach to genetic counseling begins with establishing a therapeutic alliance and engaging in an interaction that exceeds common contracting practices. The counselor establishes a sincere interest in learning about the client, what the client knows already, and what the client expects from the session. Ideally the relationship is laid down as a partnering between the counselor and the client as they negotiate their course. The exchange is guided by the client's needs and priorities yet steered by the counselor. Encouraging clients to share their relevant experiences, beliefs, and values creates the opportunity for them to convey the ways they have made meaning of their circumstances related to a condition or risk in the family. During the discussion, the counselor can assess how much the client already knows about the circumstance and how the risk or condition has affected her or him. To get a sense of how this exchange may feel, imagine you are at a family reunion and are meeting an estranged relative for the first time. To get to know her, you want to convey your respect, interest, and personal warmth and demonstrate your willingness to make a sincere effort to get to know her. You ask questions and attend thoughtfully to her responses. Of course this depends on the relative's willingness to engage with you. The ways you begin an alliance with a genetic counseling patient who is also a stranger is similar to meeting your relative, but with the professionalism that formalizes the interaction.

Genetic counselors who have not obtained family and medical history information prior to the visit may use the history-taking process to assess the patient's understanding of her circumstances and readiness to receive help. Given that patients are being asked personal information, this interaction can further establish the feelings of trust between client and counselor. In using open-ended questions, the counselor can assess the medical and family history through the client's lens. A shared history-taking process can further establish the relationship, particularly when the client shares personal experiences with the family condition or risk.

In prenatal counseling, prior knowledge or experience may be limited to what a referring physician told the woman to expect, what a friend or relative shared about prenatal screening, or what the couple read on the internet. In contrast, in pediatric and adult settings, patients are often experts on the condition that affects their child, themselves, or their family, yet may not be clear on what genetic counseling entails. Genetic counselors need to respect clients as experts while ensuring they understand the nature of the consultation to be effective active partners. In subspecialty clinics, patients with cancer or heart disease tend to know about their disease and health risks, but similarly may be unclear about what to expect in genetic counseling. Some patients who are aware of what genetic counseling entails may be seeking information to ensure they have not missed anything important or to confirm their understanding. Alternatively, they may not know their status and are seeking to understand their personal risk, the implications for their family members, or what a genetic test result may offer in clarifying the risk. The genetic counselor should explore these backstories early on to contour the session goals.

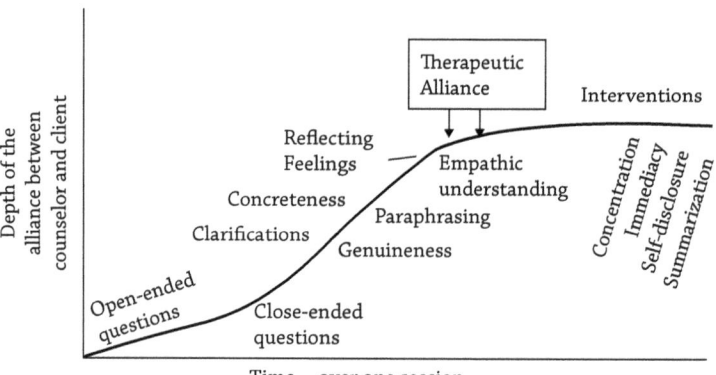

While conveying the backstory to the session, patients may share the ways that their family has discussed the risk or condition and how they have made meaning of it. At times, these explanations may be less grounded in current scientific understanding of the condition and more rooted in conveying its impact or perceived threat. Thus, use of open-ended questions can lead the counselor to develop insights into how clients are conceptualizing their risk and how they are feeling. Yet overuse of open-ended questions can suggest a disregard of the information the client has shared and jeopardize the client's trust in the counselor. Questions should become more specific and closed to yield information pertinent to the goals of the session. Counselors can follow client responses with increasingly pointed questions that indicate they are listening carefully. Counselors with keen skills learn their clients' perceptions early on as they are establishing a relationship and use them to tailor the information provided and facilitate effective decision making within the client's framework for making meaning of the risk or condition.

ASKING QUESTIONS

Counselors further shape practice dimensions by using closed-ended questions prudently, with the aim to gain a clearer understanding of the patient's relevant experiences, without unwittingly influencing the client's expression of them. Effective use of closed-ended questions that more specifically address the goal of the session reflect that the counselor is listening and responding to the client's needs. Client responses to closed-ended questions should be reflected back to convey that the counselor is seeking to understand and view the situation from the patient's perspective. When the counselor is unsure of the meaning of a client's statement, clarifications should be sought. As the counselor accumulates her understanding of the client's perspective, revisiting and confirming the session seems to be leading to the consensual goal. This effort is important to the sincerity of the relationship and can enhance the effectiveness of the session. It is often prudent to convey information relevant to the goal to inform further discussion and deliberation that follows.

PROVIDING INFORMATION

It behooves genetic counselors to identify areas where patients may want or need new information, and to teach it effectively. Genetic counseling research has shown that too often counselors verbally dominate sessions and provide information that is highly technical, abstract, and aimed at those with high literacy skills (Ellington et al. 2001; Roter et al. 2006). If counselors instead engage in a discussion or deliberation with the patients where a bit of applied and relevant information is provided, the patient is able to ask questions or explore the meaning of the information. In this way, clients are more likely to feel ownership over how they use that information to inform their choices. This approach is also consistent with how adult learners acquire new information for preference-based decision making (Epstein and Street 2007, 2011). The integration of the information provided in conjunction with establishing a counseling relationship makes up the dance that is genetic counseling. Unleashing detailed information that exceeds what the client seeks is most likely to lead to disengagement from the client and distance the counselor from achieving the session goal. Counselors should not assume that, based on their experience, they know what information and the extent of the information the client needs. There is no evidence that clients benefit from dense, detailed genetic information. Instead, there is evidence that often clients cannot follow it (Joseph et al. 2017).

When genetic counseling is routinized by providing information in a standardized way, such as using a flipbook as a guide or conveying information in a scripted order, the counseling is not relationally based (Box 8.1). Although well intended, counselors using this "standard" may deliberately, or inadvertently, ignore their client's unique perspective and assume that all clients need the same information, delivered in the same way. Adult education evidence indicates that adults learn best by relating new information to what they already know. Genetic counselors with strongly held beliefs about the specific information to be conveyed to clients to make decisions about genetic screening or testing fail to appreciate and respect

---

Text Box 8.1

Some institutions have clinical protocols that genetic counselors are supposed to follow when relaying specific genetic information. If you encounter this where you work, we encourage you to approach your administration to question the source of evidence that supports such protocols (they do not exist), or the evidence that all clients need the same information (evidence indicates a need for small amounts of tailored information). As an evidence-based alternative, propose three to five essential bits of information that you would not want any client to leave without understanding. Use the situation as an opportunity to establish a strong tie with the administration to support their need to ensure that patients get what they need, but negotiate realistic, and pertinent protocols. If there is an NSGC practice guideline related to the subspecialty, suggest that be used as the clinical protocol.

patients' prior experiences, current understanding, values, and beliefs, and the limitations of a purely scientific explanation of the risks. Further, experimental research in social psychology demonstrates that decision making is influenced by many factors, some of them irrational, that reflect common ways adults process probabilistic information. This includes use of heuristics (www.verywellmind.com/what-is-a-heuristic-2795235).

Much of a genetic counseling session is spent providing relevant information, checking for understanding, and active listening by the counselor. Key to this exchange between client and counselor is ensuring that relevant information is understood in a way that the client can use and that furthers the client's ability to make an informed decision or manage a situation that does not include a decision. During this interaction, the counselor has a responsibility to equip clients to use the information in realizing their goal. As such, the counselor should avoid assuming that the information is understood and should check in with the client to see how well the information was assimilated as relevant to the client's situation. This can be achieved by simply stating that it is important for the counselor to appreciate how the client is making sense of the information. The counselor can ask the client to reflect on the information as it is relevant to the decision or circumstance. That reflection often reveals client understanding. Checking for understanding in health communication research has been shown to be an effective way to enhance information retrieval (Ubel, Scherr, and Fagerlin 2018). If a lack of understanding or a misunderstanding is revealed, the counselor can work further with the client to improve it.

Success in communicating novel information is achieved when (1) the information is uncomplicated, specific, and repeated and (2) the counselor avoids jargon and checks for understanding. Inundating clients with information routinely fails to uphold the respect and regard for clients that is a key part of relational counseling. In contrast, a more personalized way of sharing pertinent information within a trusting relationship empowers clients to make informed choices that reflect their personal values and beliefs and will lead to fewer regrets.

RESPONSIVE DIMENSIONS

Genetic counseling aims to elicit information so that the counselor can understand clients' risk perceptions and, if appropriate, enhance their understanding. As clients respond to novel information, they are sizing up the degree of threat. Clients often seek validation of their feelings as they appraise the threat to their health. Counselors may reinforce examples shared by clients about overcoming past challenges or assess the assets that they have to manage the new threat.

Well into the relationship, after relevant information has been discussed and responded to and clients have initially appraised the threat, higher-level skills may be used by the counselor in partnership with the client to achieve the desired session goal. Paraphrasing is an important skill; it involves summarizing the client's responses or current perspective and adding an interpretation to help the client gain insight into how he or she is making meaning of the information. Paraphrasing requires advanced listening skills by the counselor, as the addition of an interpretation or insight is based on what the counselor "heard" from the client but was unspoken. It can be challenging to learn to use. Clients generally respond positively to this effort because paraphrasing demonstrates that the counselor is diligently attending and working to help the client without making her or his own presumptions. Used well, paraphrasing often helps clients progress in their decision-making process or coping with the information. For example, the counselor could say:

> You've stated several times that you feel unprepared to welcome this baby into the world, yet you have also shared numerous efforts you have made to arm yourself with information, meet other families, find a pediatrician and enlist the help of family and friends. It seems that while you feel skeptical of your abilities to parent this child, you have begun to demonstrate to yourselves your capabilities as responsible parents.

This may help a couple come to see that they have made strides in preparing for their affected child to be born even though they are scared and feel unprepared, as most parents do before a child arrives. It may also clarify for those who may have been doing all the "right things," while their hearts and heads were not in it, to realize that despite all their efforts, they do not feel at all prepared or able. Paraphrasing ideally does not include any judgment by the counselor; rather, when it accurately represents their perceptions, it can clarify for clients how they are feeling. As such, paraphrasing in this example does not aim to suggest that any way forward will be easy or that the parents are emotionally ready to welcome an affected baby into their lives, but it reflects that they are making concrete efforts to be prepared while still feeling unready. While these efforts may suggest to them that they can do it, this will only be true if they recognize that they have indeed made these efforts as capable parents preparing for a special-needs child. Such a clarification can help parents choose to seek out therapy or other help for those who come to appreciate that they will need help to prepare to welcome their baby.

To paraphrase effectively, a counselor depends on a safe and trusting relationship, understands how the couple is appraising their situation, absorbs and processes what the couple has shared, and accurately assesses what it means. If it is done at the start of a session, it will not be therapeutic and will not lead to client insight. It would merely be a summary of actions and it could be misconstrued by the clients as the counselor suggesting they ought to be doing certain things. Instead, paraphrasing occurs later in the session and emerges from a mutual exchange that has made clear what the clients have done to genuinely prepare themselves for what lies ahead and what worries and concerns them. It demonstrates an outcome of keen listening, client assessment, and compassion on the counselor's part and can go a long way in furthering relational counseling.

REFLECTING FEELINGS

To advance the counseling relationship beyond more cognitive responses, it is key that the counselor actively attends to clients' feelings. Reflecting recognition of feelings, stated or unstated, is critical to moving from a cognitive understanding of what clients are thinking to an affective understanding of their feelings. Reflection of feelings by the counselor also happens later in the relationship when the clients have come to appreciate that the counselor has heard their worries and concerns cognitively and moves on to acknowledge their affective meaning. While a counselor may find it useful to discuss how worried or distraught clients feel early in a session to acknowledge the circumstances, this serves a different purpose than reflecting feelings as the relationship has advanced. Early on it is a step in establishing the therapeutic alliance by genuinely acknowledging the difficult circumstances a couple may face. It is not intended to reflect back clients' feelings as a responsive dimension to the therapeutic alliance, nor would it be effective in doing so.

To reflect feelings accurately, it is important for counselors to have a repertoire of feeling words for example:

- Frightened
- Worried
- Optimistic
- Frustrated
- Angry
- Ambivalent
- Hopeful
- Energized
- Emotional

A hindrance to counseling can be as simple as having a limited "feelings" vocabulary. The more specific and nuanced the words used by the counselor in reflecting clients' feelings, the more meaningful the intervention can be. If the counselor uses broad descriptors, the effort may not advance the therapeutic relationship at all. In contrast, using more specific feeling labels may help clients appreciate the complexities of their reactions to a difficult circumstance. For example, "While you seem a bit relieved to have an answer to why you have cancer at such a young age, it also appears to be agitating you and leaves you feeling resentful and scared about your future cancer risks." Many of the feelings experienced in genetic counseling are multidimensional. People often choose to learn their risk information as that feels better than not knowing, but then often find themselves facing health risks they were not prepared for emotionally. These dual experiences are important to acknowledge, as it can be perplexing to clients who may have expected to be relieved by learning their risks but had not prepared themselves for having to cope with the worry and concern that accompany an elevated risk.

The breadth of feelings experienced by genetic counseling clients is wide, and counselors should challenge themselves to consider carefully what a client may be experiencing. Even when clients are in circumstances commonly addressed by a counselor, the way that particular client is responding is always novel due to the client's personal characteristics and life context. Counselors need to be prepared and to anticipate what may arise, while taking into account what the client is revealing and sharing. The timing for when to reflect client feelings is often most effective if it follows on from reflecting cognitive understanding of the client's thoughts through clarifications and paraphrases.

EMPATHIC UNDERSTANDING

Patterson (1975) proposes responsive dimensions of psychological counseling that pertain to genetic counseling: empathic understanding, communication of respect, therapeutic genuineness, and concreteness. Relational counseling rests on empathic understanding of the client. This should be a component of every genetic counseling session, with the caveat that many counseling sessions are limited to one-time encounters. The success of achieving empathic understanding is greater with clients who have experience with a genetic risk or condition. As such, it may not be an imperative to aim for deep empathic understanding of prenatal patients who recently learned about screening and are just starting to process their options and what they may mean for their family. Yet a woman carrying an affected fetus is a client who is similarly a relative stranger and yet in great need of empathic understanding as she navigates a life-changing choice.

Empathy builds over time. Any empathic statement offered early in a session is likely to be met with skepticism by the client as they are still strangers to the counselor who has no evidence from him or her (yet) to inform understanding of his or her feelings. Empathic understanding follows the juxtaposition of inquiry, listening, clarifying, teaching, processing, paraphrasing, and reflecting feelings. Simultaneous to this process, the counselor must convey sincerity, genuineness, and respect. These dimensions lend themselves to establishing the safety and trust that foster effective relational counseling that has at its core a therapeutic alliance.

Colloquially, "empathy" is used to mean thoughtfulness toward others. While empathic statements can be kind or even compassionate, they rarely advance the counseling relationship unless they are based on what has been shared between counselor and client. There is no shortcut to developing at an empathic understanding of a client. Empathy means understanding the thoughts and feelings of another person as if they were your own, without neglecting the "as if." Although more exacting definitions suggest that true empathy means experiencing another's situation as the person is experiencing it, psychology researchers define empathy as "the ability to sense other people's emotions, along with the ability to imagine what someone else may be thinking or feeling" (greatergood.berkeley.edu/topic/empathy/definition). To understand another necessitates attending to the degree that you can imagine being in the situation and sharing the feelings of your client.

Once an empathic connection is made, conveying empathic understanding is an advanced skill that is key to effective relational counseling. Yet it can be challenging even for skilled counselors to recognize when it has been achieved. It is unclear whether such an understanding needs to be vocalized to be acknowledged. Some therapists describe arriving at a point in the relationship where the client can "feel" that the therapist understands him or her and that this is sufficient (Rogers 1980). There may be a pause to acknowledge the moment between counselor and client or even a head nod but no vocalization. It implies that we have arrived together and are now on a common path that is so clear that it requires no validation. Other therapists believe that it is important to "check in" to confirm that the client feels fully understood. This can be done by restating the client's thoughts and feelings in a meaningful way, reiterating the intricacies of factors that are contributing to the client's current state of well-being, and soliciting confirmation from the client. Empathic understanding of the client, whether felt or expressed, is the pinnacle of relational counseling and serves as a bedrock for therapeutic interventions.

RESPECT AND GENUINENESS

Patterson's (1975) responsive dimensions that complement empathic understanding address the nature of the interactions between counselor and client. Conveying our respect for the client—valuing him or her as a capable person who is worth caring about—cannot be assumed. Respect is shown in many ways, starting with assessing what clients need at the time of meeting them. It is also conveyed in using critical listening skills and remaining open to learning what the client brings to genetic counseling. Using the client's name and acknowledging what has been shared are examples of communication skills that demonstrate respect. Paying attention to clients' feelings and vulnerabilities while withholding judgment is also respectful.

Therapeutic genuineness refers to the counselor being fully present, unguarded, and open to learning about the client. It means presenting your authentic self to the client, free of any pretense. Genuine interest, engagement and regard for clients can elevate their self-confidence and leave them feeling less vulnerable to potential judgment or criticism.

CONCRETENESS

To be concrete sounds relatively straightforward, yet use of vague or abstract language is common in counseling and obscures communication. As a therapeutic relationship develops, the counselor's use of specific language is strategic in achieving mutual understanding. To be concrete means to resist comparing the client's situation with that of other patients or generalizing that his or her thoughts or responses are often heard in the clinic or shared by other clients. This diminishes effective communication of empathic understanding.

Concreteness is practical in that it allows the counselor to stay close to the client's thoughts and feelings and offers the client opportunities to correct any misunderstandings. Concreteness can also be used to help clients focus on the specifics of the information, decision, or coping effort they are engaged in. Use of concreteness by the counselor can help to sift out aspects of the interaction that are less pertinent to the session goals.

THERAPEUTIC INTERVENTIONS

With empathic understanding and genuineness, the counselor is able to take greater risks in the session to help the client achieve the desired outcome. Clients who feel genuinely understood are more likely to be flexible if the counselor makes an effort to help that is not perceived as useful. Clients may say, "That's not what I meant; rather, I was trying to say..." This honest feedback helps the counselor to be more effective in meeting the client's needs. Counselors need to have the professional confidence to recognize this response not as a commentary on their skills but rather a sincere attempt by the client to be properly understood. The counselor should embrace this effort by the client as a compliment that he or she is a trusted partner. Corrections and clarifications offer the opportunity to better understand the client. Mutuality of effort toward a common goal happens with greater ease when clients correct counselors' interpretation of their meaning. This interactivity is a sign of commitment between partners in achieving a common goal.

Interventions to be used in the context of empathic understanding may be regarded as the action dimensions of the relationship (Patterson 1975). For example, as an intervention to aid decision making, counselors may confront clients on inconsistencies in their thoughts or feelings as an effort to help them clarify for themselves what is generating the conflict or which preference overrides the other. While confrontation may have a negative connotation, it need not. It typically occurs when a counselor is attentive and aiming to promote personal insight, self-reflection, and growth for the client. Although these outcomes may be addressed as they relate to the current situation, they also may be generalized beyond the situation at hand. High-functioning counselors confront clients more often about their assets and resources than their limitations. This can be particularly empowering for clients living with a genetic condition or parenting an affected child for whom new challenges await.

A useful example is to challenge clients who struggle to find the personal resources to cope effectively with their condition or with living at risk. Such a challenge may lead clients to take inventory of their personal resources expended and to brainstorm novel ones. This strength-based approach allows clients to help themselves through recognition of the extent of their capacities. It is an exercise that clients can return to later when they feel they have exhausted their resources. In contrast, it may lead some clients to appreciate that they are at capacity and cannot identify any resources they have in reserve—they are tapped out. This can lead to client awareness of the need to seek longer-term help. The counselor then has an opportunity to discuss seeking psychotherapy or participation in an advocacy/support group or other means of self-care so that the patient can renew or expand his or her resources.

Another intervention is use of immediacy to demonstrate how clients may feel taking a risk with a relative, for example. Immediacy refers to the here-and-now experience of a client relating to the counselor. If the client is able to disclose intimate feelings about her guilt and relief at not inheriting a *BRCA2* mutation that her mother and sister both have, but repeatedly relates her inability to discuss her mixed feelings with her husband or other relatives, the counselor may ask her how she feels right then in the session sharing her feelings. If she feels somewhat relieved or otherwise unburdened, the counselor may ask the client to consider in what ways she may feel similarly if she were to take a chance and tell her husband how she feels. This exchange may lead to exploration of the barriers to disclosing her status to her at-risk relatives and lead to enhancing her self-confidence that she can take the risk and feel closer to her mother and sister by being open with them. Again, the success of this type of intervention depends on having established an empathic connection with the client. Generally, immediacy describes engaging clients in how they are feeling in the counseling session and what that may represent related to the larger issues at hand.

Beyond confrontation and immediacy, interventions include use of self-disclosure to benefit the client. This higher-level skill similarly depends on having achieved an empathic understanding. While all counselors should be self-aware and understand when they are interacting with clients for their own needs even when they intend otherwise, it can be challenging to fully appreciate our distinct roles in counseling relationships (Seymour Kessler 1992). To a limited degree, counselors are serving their own needs in every counseling relationship. Staying cognizant of our own needs and recognizing when we are at risk of them leaking into our work at cross purposes to our clients' needs is critical to our effectiveness and professionalism. See Chapter 4 for a discussion of countertransference.

With the assumption that a counselor is keenly aware of how self-disclosure may be of use to a specific client, it can be very effective at legitimating a response to a difficult experience, or at leveling the playing field and reminding the client of shared life experiences. Most often self-disclosure is used to help a client to feel understood on a deeper level. An example is disclosing that you made different prenatal testing choices for each of your own pregnancies and, as such, you appreciate that each pregnancy is novel and may lead to a different decision by a parent. This may help to validate the client's choice if she is questioning herself for leaning toward making a different choice in her current pregnancy. Again, this is a higher-level intervention and is appropriately used only following the establishment of empathic understanding and after offering more concrete ways to validate a client's decisional leanings. It would be unwarranted at the start of the session or at any other point in a genetic counseling session without an established therapeutic relationship and clear understanding of clients and their needs.

Due to the past role of nondirectiveness in delineating genetic counseling, counselors are rightly cautious about engaging in personal discussions of any type with their clients. See Chapter 3 for a discussion of nondirectiveness. Sadly, this has helped to establish a relatively common disengaged stance by the counselor, one that has been described by Drs. Kessler and Weil as a distancing from the client (Seymour Kessler 1992; Weil 2003; Weil et al. 2006). It is key that genetic counselors understand the need to be genuine with their clients and develop the skills to recognize when self-disclosure, following an empathic connection, can be used effectively to enhance the patient's well-being, and not as a means for self-benefit.

Many counselors participate in and benefit from professional or peer supervision. This is generally done using recorded sessions to process the work in terms of its effectiveness in meeting the client's needs and where it may be improved. It is common for clinical psychologists to partake in psychotherapy to enhance their self-understanding within their professional roles with clients. Psychotherapy is a resource available to genetic counselors as well. Counselors often bring cases to supervision that include decisions to self-disclose or ones where it was considered to ensure that it was in the client's and not the counselor's best interests. These represent areas where professionals can facilitate further self-understanding.

At the end of a session, one of the most important interventions may be summarizing. This does not mean a literal recounting of the information provided or discussed nor a list of next steps and referrals. Rather, what is intended is a meaningful review of what the clients have learned about themselves, including resources they have identified, how they plan to overcome barriers, and if and when they may benefit from additional help. It should directly address the agreed-on goal for the session and review whether and how it has been realized. A strong personalized summary can reinforce clients' insights or ideas that arose and punctuate them as they relate to the decisions they thoughtfully considered. Highlighting clients' strengths and resources can help to boost their confidence in their abilities to move forward. As Dr. Kessler strongly reminded genetic counselors in 1999, it is important to be respectful, decent, thoughtful, and comforting to clients as they find their way in the face of a health threat to themselves or their child (Kessler 1999). The session summary should exemplify the empathy felt by the genetic counselor toward clients' circumstances and convey compassion for their pain and suffering as though the counselor has walked in their shoes.

SUMMARY

This chapter outlines dimensions of the relationship between genetic counselors and clients that can promote self-growth, identification of client strengths and resources, and recovery from suffering. Elements of relational counseling are presented with examples of how they may be actualized. We believe that the counseling skills presented in this chapter are essential to applying the counseling theories described in Chapter 9.

REFERENCES

Bernhardt, B. A., B. B. Biesecker, and C. L. Mastromarino. 2000. "Goals, Benefits, and Outcomes of Genetic Counseling: Client and Genetic Counselor Assessment." *American Journal of Medical Genetics* 94, no. 3: 189–97. http://www.ncbi.nlm.nih.gov/pubmed/10995504.

Eijzenga, W., N. K. Aaronson, D. E. Hahn, G. N. Sidharta, and L. E. van der Kolk. 2014. "Effect of Routine Assessment of Specific Psychosocial Problems on Personalized Communication, Counselors' Awareness, and Distress Levels in Cancer Genetic Counseling Practice: A Randomized Controlled Trial." *Journal of Clinical Oncology* 20: 2998–3004. https://doi.org/10.1200/JCO.2014.55.4576.

Ellington, Lee, Kimberly M. Kelly, Maija Reblin, Seth Latimer, and Debra Roter. 2011. "Communication in Genetic Counseling: Cognitive and Emotional Processing." *Health Communication* 26, no. 7: 667–75. https://doi.org/10.1080/10410236.2011.561921.

Epstein, R. M., and R. L. Street Jr. 2007. "Patient-Centered Communication in Cancer Care: Promoting Healing and Reducing Suffering." NIH Publication No. 07-6225. Bethesda, MD.

Epstein, R. M., and R. L. Street Jr. 2011. "Shared Mind: Communication, Decision Making, and Autonomy in Serious Illness." *Annals of Family Medicine* 9: 454–61. https://doi.org/10.1370/afm.1301.

Kessler, Seymour. 1992. "Psychological Aspects of Genetic Counseling. VIII. Suffering and Countertransference." *Journal of Genetic Counseling* 1, no. 4: 303–308. https://doi.org/10.1007/BF00962826.

Kessler, Seymour. 1999. "Psychological Aspects of Genetic Counseling: XIII. Empathy and Decency." *Journal of Genetic Counseling* 8, no. 6: 333–43. https://doi.org/10.1023/A:1022967208933.

Norcross, J. C., and B. E. Wampold. 2011. "Evidence-Based Therapy Relationships: Research Conclusions and Clinical Practices." *Psychotherapy* 48: 98–102. https://doi.org/10.1037/a0022161.

Patterson, C. H. 1975. *Relationship Counseling and Psychotherapy.* New York: Harper & Row.

Rogers, Carl. 1980. *A Way of Being.* New York: Houghton Mifflin.

Roter, D., L. Ellington, L. Hamby Erby, S. Larson, and W. Dudley. 2006. "The Genetic Counseling Video Project (GCVP): Models of Practice." *American Journal of Medical Genetics, Part C: Seminars in Medical Genetics* 142C, no. 4: 209–20. https://doi.org/10.1002/ajmg.c.30094.

Ubel, Peter A., Karen A. Scherr, and Angela Fagerlin. 2018. "Autonomy: What's Shared Decision Making Have to Do with It?" *American Journal of Bioethics* 18, no. 2: W11–W12. https://doi.org/10.1080/15265161.2017.1409844.

Veach, Patricia McCarthy, Dianne M. Bartels, and Bonnie S. LeRoy. 2007. "Coming Full Circle: A Reciprocal-Engagement Model of Genetic Counseling Practice." *Journal of Genetic Counseling* 16, no. 6: 713–28. https://doi.org/10.1007/s10897-007-9113-4.

Weil, Jon. 2003. "Psychosocial Genetic Counseling in the Post-Nondirective Era: A Point of View." *Journal of Genetic Counseling* 12, no. 3: 199–211. https://doi.org/10.1023/A:1023234802124.

Weil, Jon, Kelly E. Ormond, June A. Peters, Kathryn F. Peters, Barbara B. Biesecker, and Bonnie S. LeRoy. 2006. "The Relationship of Nondirectiveness to Genetic Counseling: Report of a Workshop at the 2003 NSGC Annual Education Conference." *Journal of Genetic Counseling* 2: 85–93. https://doi.org/10.1007/s10897-005-9008-1.

CHAPTER 9

Psychological Counseling Theories

Psychological counseling theories help us to understand people and how they respond to their circumstances. They serve to ground us in purposeful practice that capitalizes on people's strengths and resilience. Advancing the therapeutic aspects of genetic counseling belies the need for underlying theory that provides a framework to address clients' psychological states. Yet, arriving at a central theory of genetic counseling has eluded genetic counseling experts (Austin, Semaka, and Hadjipavlou 2014; Eunpu 1997; Kessler 1979; Weil 2000) as a singular theory is impractical given the broad scope of patient circumstances and needs.

In this chapter we argue that psychological counseling theories can be appropriated to guide genetic counseling practice. To this end, we review evidence-based theories that may be used in clinical practice and serve as a framework for outcomes research. Each makes a contribution to understanding genetic counseling clients from a different angle. We hold that intentional adoption of these therapeutic theories in practice will enable counselors to better meet their patients' needs.

Facing a chapter of multiple counseling theories, you may be filled with dread. You may fear that it will be repetitive of one of your undergraduate counseling psychology courses, or you may anticipate the tedium of details that accompany theory. To gain practical ideas from these theories, take them one at a time rather than reading the entire chapter through. Think over each theory and jot down the types of client cases and issues where it may apply. Then, next to each case type, think about ways you could use the approach to achieve a positive outcome for your client. Also reflect on a recent client you saw and consider how the theory could have been applied and what may have transpired differently as a result. Your notes may be redundant because theories overlap, and you can apply different theories to the same case. They are merely guides to help you select a framework for working with a client. There are multiple options and no right answers; this can be overwhelming at first but helpful over time as you come to appreciate having options. With experience you will find which theories most closely align with your counseling style and best meet your clients' needs.

We encourage you to adopt theory as a way to frame your casework. If you struggle to do so, this may be a fruitful topic to bring for peer supervision. You may come to use one theoretical approach more often than others. That one may resonate best with you or your clients. Your level of comfort with the approach will make it that much more genuine, and as such effective.

Taking a deliberate approach to this chapter will be practical and will help you escape boredom. Applying the ideas to your hypothetical or actual cases will help you achieve our hoped-for outcome—to become sufficiently familiar with each theory that you can conjure it up in your head while working with a client and use it to guide your counseling. This may feel awkward at first, and it may be easier after a case to arrive at a theoretical framework that would have helped. Reflecting on your casework in supervision is one way to hasten the prospective integration of theory into your work. Psychological counseling theory has much to teach us about human interactions and how they play out in our short-term counseling encounters, where our clients are often stressed. We hope you take this opportunity to heart.

GUIDING GENETIC COUNSELING WITH PSYCHOLOGICAL COUNSELING THEORY

Unlike in psychotherapy, where clients typically seek help to address a problem or setback, or are dissatisfied with an aspect of their life, our clients may be unclear how they may benefit from genetic counseling (Bernhardt, Biesecker, and Mastromarino 2000). Due to unfamiliarity with the practice, clients may not even know how to ask for what they need. As such, partnering with clients on a shared goal is critical to success. Given that clients attend genetic counseling for a variety of indications and face widely different circumstances (for example, repeated pregnancy loss, a child with intellectual disability, or risk for an adult-onset condition), no one theory or approach can guide genetic counseling patient care.

Counseling psychology theories have been shown to be effective and apply to many of the specific client needs addressed in genetic counseling. Adopting these theories has the additional benefit of providing frameworks for research to assess which interventions are most likely to benefit clients (Biesecker, Austin, and Caleshu 2017b). Studies of genetic counseling provide evidence of its effectiveness and can hone our understanding of the context where specific theoretical practices may be most or least beneficial to clients. In the absence of evidence, it has been argued by professional leaders that genetic counseling should be psychotherapeutic in helping clients mount the challenges of illness, loss, and vulnerability that accompany genetic risk and conditions (Austin et al. 2014; Biesecker, Austin, and Caleshu 2017a). Dr. Jehannine Austin and colleagues assert that "at its core, psychotherapy is about a helping relationship in which one person has the knowledge and skills relevant to helping another person address a problem through conversation" (Austin et al. 2014, p. 904). We concur that the American Psychological Association's working definition of psychotherapy is readily compatible with genetic counseling: " . . . the informed and intentional application of clinical methods and interpersonal stances derived from established psychological principles for the purpose of assisting people to modify their behaviors, cognitions, emotions, and/or other personal characteristics in directions that the participants deem desirable" (Norcross 1990, p. 218). This claim is supported by the psychologically intact state of most genetic counseling clients. They are capable of adapting to difficult circumstances but benefit from counseling by a well-trained professional.

The teaching role of genetic counseling is addressed not by psychotherapeutic theories, but rather by adult education theories (see Chapter 5). In genetic counseling, the teaching and counseling roles can be at cross-purposes (Kessler 1997); instead, they should be integrated and complementary. The personal factors that clients bring to counseling are their perceptions, values, beliefs, attitudes, ideas, thoughts, and feelings. These factors reflect both the degree of their understanding of genetic information and how they make meaning of the information as a potential threat to their psychological well-being and/or to their health (Biesecker et al. 2017b; Cameron et al. 2017). Patients' assimilation of the psychological threat of genetic information can result in lower self-esteem, suffering, stigmatization, and feelings of shame and guilt (Kessler 1984). Despite these negative consequences, most individuals adapt to even the most dire of circumstances addressed in genetic counseling. Over the course of your career you will witness the many ways that humans are resilient and accommodate to loss. Such healing occurs over time, and it can be hard to have this longitudinal view as patients often present with short-term stressors such as alarming health risks or time-sensitive decisions about a pregnancy. To address these threatening circumstances, genetic counseling needs to be efficiently and effectively therapeutic. This means providing clients the opportunity to maximize their interpersonal resources so they can make informed choices and effectively cope with circumstances for which there is no choice.

One counter-argument to the use of counseling theories in genetic counseling is its short-term nature. In the absence of a long-term relationship between therapist and client, there are limitations to applying theories intended for longer care. While this argument has merit, many psychotherapy theories have been successfully adapted for use in short-term practice (Lieberman and Yalom 1992; Rogers 1980). Pressure by third parties to substantiate theory with empirical evidence—specifically to demonstrate that long-term care was needed to achieve client outcomes—led to evidence that short-term theory-guided counseling is often as effective (Knekt et al. 2015, 2016). The evidence led to expansion of the availability of short-term psychological counseling. Many theorists embraced the evidence and were directly involved in adapting their approaches for use in short-term relationships, including Carl Rogers (Person-Centered) and Irving Yalom (Group Therapy). Those theories that are not as effectively used in short-term care, such as psychodynamic therapy and self-psychology, are likely less useful to guiding genetic counseling and not included here.

Theory to inform the psychotherapeutic aspects of genetic counseling can be drawn from well-established and evidence-based counseling theories. The challenges to applying them involve determining which theory may be helpful in a specific case, and why, and having the counseling skills to apply it effectively. Although a few theorists maintain the superiority of their theory in the care of clients, no theory has emerged from psychotherapy research as the most effective (Hunsley and Di Guilio 2002; Luborsky, Singer, and Luborsky 1976; Wampold 2001). Nor have studies shown that there is a hierarchy of theories in achieving positive client outcomes. Rather, evidence consistently suggests that *the quality of the therapeutic alliance between client and counselor is of utmost importance to the success of psychological counseling.* That is, studies assessing sessions that adhere to specific psychotherapy theories have demonstrated that their commonalities (i.e., the relational elements) are critical to achieving client benefit (see Chapter 8).

Your selection of a theory should complement the main goal of the genetic counseling session. To select a theory for a case, genetic counselors should explore with the client the issue or challenge to be addressed. Collaborating on ways that it may be addressed can give the counselor insights into appropriate theoretical approaches that match the client's concern. Facilitating decision making may be best achieved using cognitive-behavioral interventions, such as solution-focused approaches, while sessions to address adapting to a new diagnosis may benefit from a person-centered or existential theoretical approach.

Since no one theory applies to all genetic counseling clients, counselors with a repertoire at their fingertips can make tailored decisions about which theory may be most useful for addressing a specific client's needs. Here we present psychotherapy theories that we argue have direct application to genetic counseling. Each is best understood first as it was developed for psychological counseling and then as it applies to genetic counseling. Success of using theory depends on the quality of the relationship that results from the skills needed to establish a therapeutic alliance, and on the belief that clients are largely capable of helping themselves, and more so when the process is facilitated by expert professional guidance.

PERSON-CENTERED THEORY

The original genetic counseling faculty at Sarah Lawrence College taught the application of person-centered theory to genetic counseling students, aware that conveying genetic information was often a threat or experienced as a loss. Further, the notion of self-actualization—the will to strive to learn and become a better person—made the theory appealing as it recognized clients' inherent strengths. The introduction of person-centered therapy to genetic counseling at Sarah Lawrence contributed not only theoretical orientation but also concepts, including nondirectiveness, into genetic counseling parlance (Corsini 1989; Stern 2012) The early use of "nondirectiveness" to describe facilitating preference-based decisions linked this theory to genetic counseling practice, specifically in the prenatal setting.

Carl Rogers, the father of person-centered therapy, introduced the concept of nondirectiveness in an early iteration (Rogers 1951). However, he rejected the term in 1952 after coming to appreciate that it was unattainable due to the directive aspects of any human interaction, including psychotherapy. Yet the term was appropriated for genetic counseling to describe what was intended to be a non-proscriptive approach by counselors in prenatal decision making. Regrettably, interpretations of nondirectiveness in genetic counseling have been misconstrued as justification for keeping a distance from our clients to avoid influencing their decisions. Remarkably, this origin of nondirective genetic counseling entangled the roots of genetic counseling in a concept that was recognized to be improbable nearly seventy years ago. Despite this lasting setback for the genetic counseling profession, there is much to be gained by studying how person-centered theory beyond non-directiveness applies to many client circumstances.

Further, it is imperative to understand why distancing oneself from the client in the name of nondirectiveness thwarts the opportunity to engage in a therapeutic alliance—the basis of all counseling psychology theories.

Theoretical Concepts

Rogers (1980) was impressed with the client's ability to grow, and by the importance of the relationship with the therapist as a means to do so. Rogers's theory, developed in the 1940s, was based on humanistic psychology with an existential perspective. Rogers believed strongly in the phenomenological world of the client and the role of a caring therapist in helping the client to become his or her true self. Perhaps Rogers's greatest contribution to psychotherapy was his recognition of the power of the therapeutic relationship. Its characteristics of sincerity, genuineness, respect, and warmth were recognized to be of prime importance to positive client outcomes.

Rogers describes clients as motivated by a self-actualizing tendency to learn and grow to be better people. Person-centered theory is based on a set of beliefs that clients are trustworthy and resourceful, capable of self-understanding, and able to make strides toward living effective and productive lives. The desired outcome of person-centered therapy is that clients become empowered for personal change (Rogers 1980).

It may seem that person-centered therapy is a stretch for genetic counseling, particularly when practice may entail only one or two sessions with a client. Yet, on reflection, many of the underlying assumptions and beliefs apply to people under stress, such as those adjusting to and coping with a genetic condition or risk. Clients are inherently motivated to regain mastery and to cope effectively with their circumstances. They often come to genetic counseling looking to learn how to do so, not only to manage the medical aspects of the condition but also to discuss it within the family and to manage feelings of despair. Within genetic counseling, a therapeutic relationship can be framed using client-centered theory to help clients achieve these outcomes.

Theory Strengths

Person-centered theory has endured for decades. Process and outcomes research have demonstrated its effectiveness in a variety of settings, including group therapy and short-term applications. In more recent years, person-centered therapy has expanded to include how people obtain, possess, share, or surrender power and control over others and themselves (Rogers 1980). It has been successfully applied in the fields of education, industry, conflict resolution, and political negotiations.

Theory-Based Interventions

Counseling skills needed for person-centered therapy include conveying unconditional positive regard toward the client, engaging in a genuine approach, and achieving empathic understanding of the client. These require mature active listening and attending behaviors. Clients need to hear their own words reflected back by the counselor in a way that facilitates clarification and promotes personal insight. The counselor invites or even probes clients to share their feelings. The counselor may use confrontation to help clients recognize inconsistencies or conflicting emotions or behaviors that they were not aware of. An expert counselor can use self-disclosure as a tool to validate clients' feelings and to promote understanding in the relationship. These interventions aim to achieve a sense of empathic connection between counselor and client. When clients feel truly understood, they can often take the next steps to cope with the genetic risk or loss.

Application to Genetic Counseling

A therapeutic relationship between genetic counselor and client is of critical importance in facilitating client coping, adaptation, and personal growth. Without a relationship built on trust, even the teaching component of counseling is likely to be ineffectual. The counselor needs to create a permissive and accepting climate for the relationship to develop. Use of tools to establish a level of client comfort in sharing personal information and intimate feelings is key. Clients appreciate being regarded as valued and capable by the counselor and, as such, can work toward making personal meaning of genetic information. The stress from a health threat, such as a genetic risk or diagnosis, may inhibit learning information or result in feeling out of control. Addressing clients' psychological distress can help them identify resources for addressing their needs.

For example, if a counselor has established a therapeutic relationship with a client and difficult news follows, such as the presence of an expanded repeat in the HTT gene, designating the eventuality of Huntington disease, the client may feel sufficiently safe to express his deep concerns. He may be worried whether his marriage will endure his future condition. The counselor can explore with the client how the couple has managed past struggles and probe the client for examples of when he found strength in the relationship he hadn't previously appreciated. Reminders of his resilience may ease some of the initial distress that accompanies such difficult news. Not all marriages have the resources to survive such difficulties. Within a trusting relationship, the patient may be able to find the strength to follow up with couples therapy to anticipate and prepare for the challenges that lie ahead. Within a therapeutic connection with a genetic counselor, a client is more likely to actively participate in making a decision to pursue follow-up psychotherapy to address such major life issues. The client's willingness to share such a vulnerability with the genetic counselor, and the counselor's acceptance of the client's significant concerns, can lead the client to feel empowered to seek further help.

Many parents of children with delayed development or a chronic illness describe experiences where they felt isolation and shame (Lipinski et al. 2006). During phases of adaptation, such as appraising the situation, parents reflect on the uncertainties and unfamiliarity of their circumstances (Lazarus and Folkman 1984; Rosenthal, Biesecker, and Biesecker 2001). They often express perceptions that their circumstances are so rare that they feel isolated and without social resources. Person-centered approaches aimed at recognizing and acknowledging these appraisals may be useful to help clients identify adaptive coping strategies and sources of social support. Conveying understanding of clients' feelings to the degree that they can recognize their ability to move forward with their lives is another potential application of person-centered theory. Ideally, person-centered genetic counseling interactions lead to gains in personal insight that carry over into other aspects of a client's life. In this way, genetic counseling can contribute to a client's personal growth and serve as an agent of personal change and enhanced strength.

COGNITIVE-BEHAVIORAL THEORIES

In contrast to person-centered theory, cognitive-behavioral therapy (CBT) theories represent a diversity of approaches. Generally, they are based on a structured learning model developed by Ellis in the 1950s, the underlying premise being that there are reciprocal interactions among cognitions, behaviors, and emotions (Ellis 1957). Within the context of CBT, psychological distress is approached as a function of disturbances in cognitive processes.

Theoretical Concepts

CBT aims to help clients accept that they make mistakes yet have the opportunity to learn from them. The focus is on changing cognitions to produce desired changes in affect and behavior. Clients are viewed as the agents of change, while the therapist guides them to alternative ways of thinking about the problem and its potential solutions.

Theory Strengths

CBT involves interventions for targeted problems with practical outcomes. These techniques have been used in group therapy, couples therapy, family therapy, and individual therapy. CBT has been adapted successfully to many contexts, including health care. Short-term models, such as problem-solving or solution-focused interventions, have withstood the rigors of research. The general aim of all of these approaches is for clients to learn strategies to solve dilemmas that can be applied to other situations in their lives, so, similar to the goals of person-centered theory there can be long-term positive results.

CBT therapists are exceptional listeners. They attend to faulty or distorted thinking and direct clients to approaches to change them. This is done by disputing thoughts through exploring the evidence behind them, or by assigning homework that contributes to self-evaluation and change. For example, clients may be assigned the task of changing their language to get rid of the "oughts" and the "shoulds." CBT therapists frequently use humor, particularly to confront exaggerated thinking. Interventions include the use of imagery, where clients are asked to imagine their worst or most inappropriate feelings and to experience them intensely, then to change the experience to alter their feelings. The goal of these interventions is to change the client's ways of thinking in order to evoke positive change in self-image or realistic self-assessments that can be sustaining.

Application to Genetic Counseling

Genetic counseling clients frequently present with a dilemma or a choice. CBT interventions can be used with either (Biesecker et al. 2017a). Even without formal training in cognitive techniques, prenatal genetic counselors can use a strategy that engages the clients in creating "pro" and "con" lists, a technique borrowed from CBT, when they are uncertain about undergoing testing. Counselors can then explore with clients their reasons for their attitudes toward testing and whether they are consistent with what they value about the information and the decision at hand. This shared approach can lead to informed decision making where clients are less likely to regret their decision.

Clients most often make decisions based on the anticipated outcomes of a test. As such, when counseling a couple who is ambivalent about prenatal testing, the genetic counselor may ask the partners to participate in a thought exercise. To consider the impact of the outcomes, the counselor would ask them to imagine that they chose not to undergo testing and that the fetus is diagnosed with a condition. Clients are asked to rehearse what their reactions may be. The next step is to contrast them to their anticipated responses to undergoing testing and learning that the fetus has a condition. While it is challenging for people to anticipate how they would feel in an unlikely hypothetical future, this visual imagery strategy helps clients increase their awareness of their likely responses. Couples can be helped to discover which decisional consequence may be less difficult to endure. This example illustrates how CBT interventions can be used to actively engage clients who are considering prenatal testing. Such interventions can engage clients in a process that leads to informed decisions and is less likely to result in decisional regret.

Other situations where CBT can be effectively applied in genetic counseling is when clients are inconsistent, saying one thing and doing another, or thwarting their own stated personal values. Clients are often unaware of their inconsistencies, and pointing them out can facilitate personal insight into competing thoughts or feelings. With exploration, clients may be helped to understand more about their true thoughts or feelings about the situation at hand. This approach can also be useful in working with couples who have a difference of opinion—for example, about whether to undergo genetic testing.

The counselor may reframe for the client cognitive distortions or unrealistic thinking. Reframing provides a new perspective from which clients can view their thoughts or feelings. A client overwhelmed and conflicted when given the choice whether to undergo prenatal testing may be asked how she would feel if she had no choice. This reframes the issue in a way that those who value perceived control will likely find themselves better able to view the choice as an opportunity and settle into making it. For those who wish there was no choice, they may be helped to accept that they can decline the choice and proceed with the pregnancy accordingly.

Behavior modification, a specific type of CBT intervention, also has application in genetic counseling. If parents are seeking help in keeping their child with a metabolic condition on a restricted diet, the genetic counselor can teach them behavior-modification techniques to help their child. Behavior modification may also be used as an educational intervention for children with attention or behavior problems. While genetic counselors less frequently have occasion to teach patients behavior modification, those who work in pediatrics may find a variety of CBT interventions helpful to parents.

PROBLEM-SOLVING THEORY

Problem-solving or solution-focused therapy falls within the broader category of CBT but is sufficiently relevant to genetic counseling that it deserves specific attention. Solution-focused approaches originally were based on the concept that fostering clients' ability to solve a problem was more important than understanding the problem's root (Berg 1994). This idea was coupled with CBT approaches and used to develop techniques for helping clients improve their ability to solve problems. In the 1980s deShazer and colleagues changed the focus to identifying solutions (de Shazer 1985). Several different models of brief problem-solving or solution-focused therapy exist and have demonstrated their effectiveness. Clients can also use solution-focused strategies in other areas of their lives as a sustaining benefit of these approaches.

Theoretical Concepts

Use of problem-solving theory to guide counseling respects clients' ability to solve their own problems. The therapist strives to understand not the problem, but rather the client's perceptions of its consequences and potential solutions. The client is regarded as the expert in understanding the importance of the problem and as the source of the solutions. It draws on the resourcefulness and strengths of clients and is often creative.

Theory Strengths

Problem-solving approaches are rapid and efficient. They fit into the lives and resources of many clients. Most clients seek therapy because they are unhappy with something in their life and would like to change it. Problem-solving therapy capitalizes on this motivation. Clients also appreciate concrete evidence that they achieved an outcome from therapy.

The educational slant to problem-solving therapy provides clients with an approach to consider using when future problems arise, thus minimizing the need for subsequent visits. There are extensive uses of problem-solving therapy, from self-help groups to health care decision making, including genetic counseling.

Theory-Based Interventions

Problem-solving therapy begins with the identification of a problem, worry, or concern. Clients offer a narrative of their experience to provide the context for the problem. In certain problem-solving approaches, clients can be taught contrasts between emotion-focused coping strategies and task-focused coping strategies. Clients benefit from learning that emotion-focused strategies work best with problems that cannot be changed, and task-focused strategies aim to change or modify the problem. Research suggests that those who employ both strategies appropriately to different types of stressors adapt best (Lazarus and Folkman 1984).

After identifying and describing the problem, clients may be asked to brainstorm potential solutions to the problem. They are asked to free associate so that even seemingly outrageous solutions are noted. Once a list is generated, then the client may be asked to discuss the short- and long-term consequences of each of the potential solutions. These consequences can be noted as positive or negative. Any solutions with significantly negative or non-beneficial consequences are stricken early from the list. The remaining solutions may be discussed in terms of their barriers. Some may have insurmountable barriers and as such do not offer a viable option. Once this exercise is complete, clients can rank their solutions according to those that have the most potential benefit with the least restrictive barriers. Once a solution is identified and chosen, then a plan for implementing it can be developed.

Throughout a process like the one outlined, the counselor compliments clients on their ability to come up with solutions and work to identify the one most likely to be successful. Offering positive reinforcement is one of the strategic factors in solution-focused therapy. The therapist can also facilitate the client's understanding of a problem by using techniques such as scaling. Clients may be asked to rank their feelings about a problem or potential solution on a scale of 1 to 10. This may also be done using a visual analog scale. Alternatively, the client may be asked to envision what an ideal outcome of the problem might look like. This has been referred to as the "miracle question." It allows clients to have a vision of what they are striving to achieve. Solution-focused counseling may also employ use of the "empty chair" role-play where clients rehearse with the counselor how they might discuss a difficult issue with a family member. As these examples suggest, solution-focused therapy offers a number of interventions that may be useful in genetic counseling.

Application to Genetic Counseling

Short-term decision making in genetic counseling is well suited to a problem-solving approach. Decisions about screening tests, diagnostic tests, predictive tests, or carrier tests may be deliberated in the context of obstacles. If a solution-focused approach is taken, the client's coping skills in adapting to a diagnosis or its implications can be honed to become more effective.

Clients often bring practical problems to the genetic counseling session. For example, parents may ask when and how they should tell their daughter about her diagnosis of Turner syndrome. There are no "right" answers to these types of questions, and the best advice we can offer parents is most often their own. Rather than offering answers, a genetic counselor can apply a solution-focused approach to help clients realize that they have the capacity and ideas to answer their own question. Parents have certainly considered over the years when the best time would be and how they should discuss the diagnosis with their daughter. A solution-focused intervention can help them anticipate how to overcome certain obstacles or find ways to manage their own fears. Asking them how they would ideally like the conversation to go may provide them with a goal to shoot for, and then plans may be formulated to accomplish it. There are practical examples of challenges or problems clients seek to overcome in all practice settings. As such, problem-solving and solution-focused theories have much to offer, including concrete interventions that can be implemented without further training.

FEMINIST THEORIES

Feminist theories cover a broad range of approaches that have a strong sociopolitical heritage. The feminist theories were born from a strong reaction against not only psychoanalytic theory, but many theories that were identified as paternalistic or male-generated. Feminist theories capitalize on women in relationship to others. Research has demonstrated that women define themselves through their relationships and that their worldviews involve the role and importance of these relationships (Gilligan 1989; Miller 1976). As such, theories of feminist therapy promote relational issues in the context of family and community. Such theories accommodate the needs of clients who come from disparate backgrounds and various ethnocultural backgrounds.

Theoretical Concepts

Feminist therapists promote the importance of self-awareness and often share their personal/professional biases or values with clients. Such self-disclosure is an acknowledgment of the humanness of the therapist and her commitment to engage in a mutual relationship with the client. An important goal of most feminist theories is the restoration of client power, so it is not uncommon to hear them described as empowerment therapies. This descriptor is reminiscent of their roots in the 1960s women's movement in the United States and is consistent with the social reform of that time and the contemporary resurgence of women's power.

Theory Strengths

Feminist theories broadened the opportunities for women to benefit from psychotherapy. Women increasingly became therapists, studied women's issues, and developed theories specific to women. Female psychotherapists accordingly served as role models for female clients. The broad context in which a woman's life is considered in feminist therapy provides multiple opportunities for application of gained skills. For example, the approach may include involving a partner or best friend in psychotherapy for a short time, or even an important member of the woman's community. This recognizes the bidirectional nature of relationships and the shared responsibility for reinstilling power to the woman that will carry over when she reengages in her community. These theories have been practiced as group therapy, couples therapy, and family systems therapy.

Theory-Based Interventions

Feminist therapy varies widely. The interventions are more nebulous than those of other theories presented in this text. Generally, self-awareness techniques are used by feminist therapists. Therapists often begin by asking clients to tell their story, as the narrative is an important aspect of the therapeutic process. It sets the scene for understanding the context of the woman's life, and in particular her significant relationships. Thus, feminist therapists use active listening skills and strive to develop an empathic connection with their clients. Therapists may use self-disclosure and confrontation as ways to help clients learn more about themselves. Positive reinforcement is used to help women recognize and use their inherent strengths. Specific techniques to promote self-discovery include writing or journaling, artistic expression, and role-playing. Women may be asked to listen and discover new dimensions of themselves within their relationship with the therapist.

Assertiveness training, a more psychoeducational intervention, has its roots in feminist theory and aims to support women in caring for themselves, speaking up for their own needs, and making positive change in their lives. Similar techniques have been applied to the field of conflict resolution, where women are empowered to advocate for themselves in a constructive manner.

Application to Genetic Counseling

The majority of genetic counselors are women and many clients are also women, particularly in prenatal and cancer genetic counseling contexts. As such, feminist approaches have much to offer genetic counseling. In the prenatal diagnostic clinic, many of the issues are particular to women as they carry the developing baby. There may be physical changes or concerns about the pregnancy itself or about past pregnancy losses. Similarly, many aspects of impending parenthood pertain to women's needs and concerns. Women may have concerns about their marriage or their ability to parent. They may choose to share issues of sexual intimacy or infidelity. Feminist approaches empower women to share the issues that are important to them. Prenatal diagnosis counseling presents an opportunity to address these issues and help clients assess whether further counseling with a psychotherapist is indicated. To assess the issues efficiently, the genetic counselor must listen carefully to the woman's story and help her prioritize her greatest source of concern as it relates to the goal of the genetic counseling session. Ideally, the genetic counselor would partner with the client on how she wants to address her concern and an approach is negotiated. Genetic counselors can validate women's concerns, discuss their origins, address their worries, and help to identify their resources for coping with distress. The genetic counselor can connect with the client in a manner that engenders trust and through which the counselor can convey positive messages about the client's successes. This can be an empowering experience for the genetic counseling client. In an exploratory outcome study of genetic counseling, clients and counselors noted the importance of feeling connected to one another and, for the client, feeling understood (Bernhardt, Biesecker, and Mastromarino 2000).

Another application of feminist therapy to genetic counseling is in breast and ovarian cancer counseling, where women's issues abound. Many of the issues for women in cancer risk clinics are about their relationships with relatives or their partners. They may have unresolved grief issues related to a mother or sister who has died that may contribute to their own cancer worries. Women often share worries about dying and leaving their children. The cancer risk information that is provided has personal meaning that is embedded within these relationships. Feminist therapy offers a useful framework for counseling women in these settings. Explicit examples are clients with a *BRCA 1* pathogenic variant facing choices about prophylactic surgery. Women often seek to feel empowered to make good decisions for themselves about their life and their health that relate to aspects of what it means to be a woman.

GROUP THERAPY

Most theories of psychotherapy can be applied as group therapy. There are characteristics of group therapy central to its effectiveness that cut across theoretical frameworks. The basis of its success lies with the interpersonal relationships established within the group (Yalom 2005). As such, the central premise of group therapy is that the members interact at a level that approaches co-counseling. It is the group members' relationships and the processes that constitute the intervention that lead to personal change, while the therapist acts primarily as a skilled facilitator. Outcomes research has demonstrated the success of group therapy in a number of different settings and with a wide range of clients.

Theoretical Concepts

Common factors among therapy groups distinguish them from self-help or educational groups. These factors originate from research into long-term group therapy, but many have been achieved in short-term groups as well. Yalom (2005) identified eleven therapeutic factors central to the process of personal change achieved through group therapy: instillation of hope, universality, imparting information, altruism, corrective recapitulation of the family group, development of socializing techniques, imitative behavior, interpersonal learning, cohesiveness, catharsis, and existential factors. Not all of these factors contribute to every group or every member's growth, but when analyzing the elements of the process that contribute to the desired outcomes, they lie among these factors.

Most groups share a central issue that brings the members together. The therapist plays an important role in determining this issue or the reason for bringing the group together. As groups begin, the therapist contracts with participants to create "rules of conduct" that protect people's privacy and respect their role as active group participants. Members are reminded of the need to listen as well as to share, and therapists encourage those who are more hesitant to participate and discourage those who tend to dominate the discussion. As the group's dynamics mature, these efforts tend to be taken on by group members. The group members develop a process that involves helping each another as they help themselves. The group represents a slice of larger society and may serve as a representation of the participants' roles in relation to others or as a transition into a larger community. It is a remarkably powerful experience to participate in or to facilitate a group and is a therapeutic approach that has promise for genetic counseling.

Theory Strengths

The versatility of group therapy, its staying power, and its ability to stand up to the rigors of research demonstrate its universality. It shares an advantage over other forms of therapy by serving as a microcosmic experience that can model the client's presence in a family or a larger sociocultural context. And it capitalizes on people's strengths.

Theory-Based Interventions

A group therapist has expertise with a theoretical framework and with group process. Facilitation is a key role for the leader, who should be highly flexible and creative. Group therapists are particularly good listeners who attend not only to the literal interpretation of what is said but also the underlying meaning and intent, and to the members' responses. They are empathic and serve as important role models to participants who become empathic of one another. An additional intervention used by therapists is to provide role modeling for members through use of effective self-disclosure. Therapists may have to engage in conflict management or to renegotiate roles within the group to facilitate the process. This may be accomplished through use of questioning, confrontation, alignment, and paradox. Many therapeutic interventions lend themselves well to the group process and are selected by therapists according to their theoretical orientation and experience, and the needs of the group.

Application to Genetic Counseling

Group genetic counseling for a wide variety of indications may be offered by a genetic counselor who has undergone training on group process. A group addressing bereavement for parents who have chosen to terminate a pregnancy, who have lost a stillborn child, or who have endured pregnancy losses or infertility, or whose child died of a genetic condition may be transformative for these parents. These shared experiences have direct parallels with parent support groups, which genetic counselors may also help to organize or facilitate. Delineating the difference between group therapy and support groups is important. Support groups are often psychoeducational and rely on providing information and informal social support. Professionals may be involved to facilitate the development of support groups and to promote peer leadership. Genetic counselors may remain involved and continue to support the active participation of group members but do not play a central role in the group process to facilitate the personal growth of members.

Genetic counselors who serve as leaders of group therapy groups ought to have training in group process and familiarity with the circumstances that brought the group together. They are ideally suited to lead groups that include members who have been through the same novel circumstances that may be less familiar to a social worker or psychologist. Having expertise in the science of the tests or the condition that brought members together allows for the provision or clarification of information when appropriate. Genetic counselors also may bring to the group their own professional experiences working with many individuals who have been in similar circumstances.

In groups that are established to promote personal growth or adaptation, the group is structured to resemble psychotherapy groups. Clients may join a group because, for example, they have endured a life tragedy or face a difficult health risk and feel very isolated by the circumstances.

In the process of adapting, clients seek to make meaning of their circumstances—struggling to understand why it happened (metaphysically), identifying ways to manage their distress, and regaining a sense of mastery or control over their lives. As such, with additional training, group therapy offers ways for genetic counselors to expand their expertise and reach. They can fill a unique niche for clients who have sought out psychotherapy but found therapists hesitant to take on a group due to their lack of familiarity with the circumstances and content members are likely to be addressing.

FAMILY THERAPY THEORIES

Family therapy emanated from a broad range of theories that in the 1960s and 1970s represented a significant shift from theories of individual psychotherapy. These theories hold that individuals are best understood in the context of their relationships and interactions within the family. The family is viewed as an interactive system where a change in one part results in a change to other parts. Family therapy provides a context for understanding how individuals function in relationship to and with other members. The premise of the majority of these theories is that to produce change in individual members related to the problem, the whole family must engage together in a therapeutic intervention. Specific aims often are to help family members recognize relationships or patterns of communication that are dysfunctional in an effort to establish new modes of interacting that reduce psychological distress and are more effective.

Theoretical Concepts

The focus of most family theories is on patterns of communication. For example, patterns of communication that aim to control family members are seen as dysfunctional. Beyond communication, family therapy has been applied to problems of marital distress, estrangement, helping members to realize their potential, or poor family functioning.

Key constructs addressed in family therapy include enmeshment (the failure of individuals to appropriately differentiate from each other), triangulation of relationships, power coalitions, family rules that govern communication patterns, and family-of-origin dynamics. Most family therapists have training in family context and systems.

Theory Strengths

Working with the family system offers an enhanced perspective on understanding and working through both individual problems and relationships. There may be challenges in achieving commitment and involvement from all family members in therapy sessions. Yet, the importance of family context in many ethnocultural groups suggests that these theories may offer one of the most important orientations for working with individuals from certain ethnocultural backgrounds.

Theory-Based Interventions

Family communication patterns are often a focus of these theories as they represent some of the underlying relational issues and power differentials. In healthy families, individuals are encouraged to express their thoughts and feelings with few rules or restrictions, even when they differ with family members. Beyond communication interventions, family therapy offers clients understanding of important parameters in healthy family relationships. Hierarchies between parents and children are important to maintain as well as differentiation among individuals that is developmentally appropriate.

Application to Genetic Counseling

The process of genetic counseling often includes discussion of family communication, relationships, and functioning, reflecting central targets in family therapy. These family characteristics suggest that the use of family therapy techniques may enhance the effectiveness of genetic counseling. The threat of passing on a condition from parent to child, or one sibling being identified to be at high risk for disease while the other is not, raises threats to family relationships. This is not only because genetic conditions may be transmitted in families, but also because illness or living at risk affects all family members. Even the option of undergoing genetic testing is a family affair, as one person's decision to undergo predictive testing may reveal information about another family member. Further, the life-altering choices that some genetic counseling clients face often impact the entire family.

Constructing a family pedigree is not dissimilar from constructing a genogram, a tool grounded in family therapy that considers family communication and dynamics. Several genetic counselors have suggested a role for constructing genograms in genetic counseling (Daly et al. 1999; Eunpu 1997; Peters et al. 2006). This expansion of the family history offers a platform for adding information that can be used to help individuals anticipate how information may be received or used within a family. With a hybrid family tool, the counselor can refer to past patterns of communication in helping the client anticipate future ones, when assessing the family's ability to absorb new health-threatening information.

Awareness of healthy parameters and boundaries in relationships allows genetic counselors more confidence in assessing areas of family dysfunction. Experience shows that enmeshment with an ill child or power struggles between teens with a chronic illness or disability seeking their independence and their parents, would not be unexpected in a genetic counseling encounter. The concepts of family theories can be used to empower genetic counselors to recognize family dysfunction or sources of distress and can in turn enhance the effectiveness of genetic counseling at working within existing dynamics. If genetic counseling clients share that they are seeking relief from chronic family dysfunction, referral to a family therapist is indicated.

For example, a mother seeks to have her young children undergo carrier testing for a condition that may be passed on to the next generation. In the counseling session, it becomes apparent that it is the mother who seeks this information to relieve her guilt and the uncertainty about her children's status. In this case, the genetic counselor may use family therapy techniques to help the mother understand that the outcome of testing may not provide either. If her children are carriers, she may experience even more guilt and new uncertainty related to whether they will have affected children. Further, if she authorizes carrier testing, her children would be stripped of the opportunity to choose not to know their carrier status as adults. Some individuals may choose not to know such information in an effort to remain optimistic or hopeful that they were spared the pathogenic variant in the family. If they forgo a biological pregnancy, there may be no reason for them to learn the information. If a mother is enmeshed with her children, which can happen as an overprotective reaction to an at-risk child, she might fail to appreciate that her child may make a different choice as an adult and may earnestly believe that her own interests represent the best interests of her children. This case may sound harsh, as most families manage risk information well and support one another. But there are cases when the pain and suffering of a parent is so significant that it affects relationships and can lead to disempowerment of adult children.

STRENGTH-BASED COUNSELING

A contemporary counseling theory with important implications for genetic counseling is strength-based counseling (Smith 2006). This approach to psychotherapy seeks to understand human virtues and to determine what strengths a person has used to effectively deal with life. It may be thought of as asset building. It emphasizes the benefits of human diversity and recognizes cultural and social groups as sources of strengths. As such, this approach has been successfully used in working with clients from many backgrounds and ethnocultural groups.

Strengths develop from a dynamic, contextual process that is rooted in the client's culture. This approach is based on the understanding of humans as self-righting. Strengths often explored in psychotherapy are courage, insight, optimism, perseverance, perspective, and purpose in life.

Theory-Based Concepts

In lieu of a theoretical framework, there are stages of strength-based counseling: creating a therapeutic alliance, identifying strengths, assessing presenting problems, encouraging and instilling hope, framing solutions, building strength and confidence, empowering, changing, building resilience, and evaluating. Given the nascent nature of strength-based counseling, no evidence yet exists on its effectiveness.

Application to Genetic Counseling

Given that most genetic counseling clients are adapting to health-threatening genetic information rather than seeking therapy to address a major personal problem, most have the resources to manage the stress. Even those found to be in high-risk situations can be helped to find courage, hope, and empowerment. The positive frame of a theoretical approach conveys respect and trust that clients can manage the risk or other hardship that has come their way. The positive frame of a strength-based approach dwells not on the threat of the information, but rather on the resources available to manage it. It is uplifting for clients to identify ways they already have the internal, and often external, resources to manage, even if it will be challenging to do so. Its appeal lies in capitalizing on clients' agency and abilities, a hopeful approach that can be uplifting to counselors as well as clients.

CRISIS COUNSELING

Genetic information can create a crisis for clients. When they learn unexpected or particularly difficult news, they often instinctively and subconsciously "shut down" as a means of self-protection. Defense mechanisms subsequently engage to shield the person from the full realization and impact of devastating information. How a crisis "looks" varies widely. Think of videos of victims of violence, abuse, neglect, war, and atrocities. They may cry out in pain, turn silently inward, get up and leave, or become nonresponsive. These contrasting responses illustrate that it is often hard to recognize when our patients are in a crisis. Similarly, they are often unable to recognize or articulate what is happening to them.

There are ways to identify a crisis nonetheless. The first clue is the circumstances—delivery of unexpected and seriously threatening news. For example, a mother may learn that her child has a pathogenic variant in a gene that predisposes to a neurodegenerative disorder that was included on a panel of genes for retinal disease. When testing is done to investigate the cause of retinal disease, the neurodegenerative conditions on the panel are discussed with parents, but they are rare and unlikely to occur. Based on the retinal changes that prompted testing, the identification of a pathogenic variant amounts to unexpected presymptomatic testing for an untreatable neurodegenerative condition of childhood. The news is shocking and devastating. The parents would be expected to experience a crisis in response to this information.

Characteristics of a crisis include the inability to think clearly and thus to respond to questions. Some patients ask the same questions repeatedly. Others may disengage entirely or sit rigidly and appear stone-faced. Unfortunately, these patients or parents are often described by health care providers as "in denial." This is a misnomer for the human instinct to engage defense mechanisms that blunt one's thoughts, feelings, and actions. They heard the news and are not denying it, but taking in the full meaning is too cognitively and affectively painful to bear. Human defense mechanisms engage to protect our psyches and our hearts.

Strategies for working with parents or patients in crisis are practical (France 2014; Koocher, Curtiss, and Patton 2001). Do not make demands of those in crisis. Answer questions (repeatedly if needed), witness their pain, accompany them, reassure them (realistically), use kind words, and give them private personal space if they recognize they need it. If your patients in crisis traveled by car, ensure that someone drives them home to keep them safe. Leave them with your contact information, and that of a social worker or therapist, and relay plans for the next time you will meet with written information about what will happen at that time. Assume they will remember none of what you convey and take responsibility for being directive in leading them safely home into the arms of their loved ones. Call them in a couple of days to check in.

Genetic counselors who are accustomed to providing client-centered care often find crisis work challenging as it demands taking control, steering patients, and telling them what to do. All these actions are counselor initiated and quite directive. Crisis training can provide further compassionate strategies that do not ask much of clients. Most crises are time-limited, and as patients are able to begin to absorb the devastating news, they will seek information, reassurance, and options in their own time. Be there when they have emerged and are ready, but do not attempt to provide this information prematurely. Avoid describing your patients as "in denial."

Importantly, none of the psychotherapeutic theories reviewed in this chapter can be applied to care for parents or patients in crisis. Participation in a therapeutic alliance necessitates clients' access to and articulation of feelings and thoughts. Theoretically based counseling can be used to help as people emerge from a crisis, but not as they are experiencing one. One of the biggest clues that a patient is in crisis is his or her inability to engage in meaningful exchange. This should not be mistaken for not caring, or dismissal of the information; rather, this behavior reflects subconscious efforts to keep suffering at bay. Further, do not be fooled by those who appear cognitively intact and who take charge and demand information (but do comply). Keep in mind the many "faces" of a crisis and recognize that this pattern can occur even among those who have "shut down." This is a less common response in a crisis, but people who instinctively fall back on a pattern of solving the problem may also attempt to do so in a crisis. Yet they too are incapable of processing their responses, and you will have to engage them again at a later time when they can access their personal resources.

One mother of a newborn diagnosed with trisomy 18 shortly after birth asked the same questions about her baby over and over for several hours. She could not retain the information nor recall that she had asked the questions prior. Her efforts secured her the company of a genetic counselor during a time of acute suffering with the inability to otherwise relate. Never abandon patients in time of need, regardless of your inability to meet their needs. Recognize a crisis, but remember that the next one is likely to look quite different and use the circumstances as your main clue to understanding what is transpiring.

BEREAVEMENT COUNSELING

Bereavement counseling is specific to addressing loss. It is best offered when patients or clients have had a bit of time to weather the initial pain and sorrow of their loss. The counseling is atheoretical and focuses primarily on ways to promote healing and help patients find ways to look forward to the future again (Parkes and Prigerson 2009; Worden 2008). Grieving is a very personal process and one that people largely figure out for themselves. Scholars differentiate people as those who tend to be instrumental versus intuitive grievers. The former tend to keep busy, distract themselves, and take action to move their lives forward, while the latter tend to engage in more cerebral and private processes that rely on their instincts for what will help them to heal. The latter tend to seek ways to understand and respond to the suffering as a way to recover. Many of these responses come naturally; although they can be learned, they are generally innate.

In genetic counseling, there is much loss and suffering among our patients and their parents. Counselors may be present at the time of death but are more often engaged with clients who are working to heal from their loss. Much of the work involves active listening and offering comfort in witnessing the pain and suffering of others. It is not formulaic, nor do patients progress linearly through stages as was once promoted. Rather, grief is a haphazard, chaotic process that is personal and often isolating. Participation in support groups, such as Compassionate Friends for parents who have lost children, can bring comfort and provide an opportunity to help others. Bereavement counseling courses are offered regularly through hospitals or local universities. These can be beneficial in familiarizing yourself with grief and approaches of value to patients. It is also important to learn the resources in your institution and community.

SUMMARY

This chapter outlines psychotherapy theories with application for genetic counseling. Each theory makes a contribution to clients in specific circumstances. Despite their distinct characteristics, theories in practice are remarkably similar. Research aimed at demonstrating that one theoretical approach is more effective than another has generally failed to identify one that is most effective. Much of current research has shown that the commonalities, primarily the relational components, are central to the efficacy of theoretically informed psychological counseling.

Becoming more familiar with these psychotherapy theories will equip you with a repertoire of ways to address the needs of your clients (Box 9.1). Keep in mind that one case may be approached from more than one psychotherapeutic theory. What might present itself as a case facilitating reproductive decision making may evolve into bereavement counseling due to a prior loss. Genetic counselors must be flexible in their approaches to clients and able to adapt to evolving circumstances or information. The most important component of any of these theoretical approaches is the establishment of the therapeutic alliance and commitment to the responsibilities that stem from that relationship.

Text Box 9.1

A pregnant woman is identified to be carrying a fetus affected with Duchenne muscular dystrophy (DMD). Her brother has DMD and her maternal uncle died of the condition. How would the counselor approach this client based on the theories discussed in this chapter?

Person-centered—The counselor focuses on her thoughts and feelings toward the pregnancy and the complexities of raising a son with DMD or terminating the pregnancy in light of her relationships with her brother and uncle.

CBT—The counselor focuses on the decision she faces about the pregnancy and her anticipation of the outcomes of both options.

Problem-solving—The counselor helps the client formulate a list of solutions beyond continuing or terminating the pregnancy, such as adopting her brother's strategies for managing his life, capitalizing on what the family has learned about DMD to date, and hope for improved treatments. Discussion also includes the barriers that limit those solutions.

Feminist—The counselor focuses on the woman's relationship with her mother and her developing baby and what her situation means not only for her but for her mother and sisters as well.

Family—The counselor focuses on the meaning of the pregnancy for all of her family and tries to understand how they are communicating about the diagnosis and how the information is anticipated to affect her brother and others in the family.

Crisis—The counselor focuses on the immediate threat of the information and the need to keep the woman safe and to follow up with her for counseling at a later time.

Bereavement—The counselor focuses on the loss she will experience with either of her options—she will lose either a wished-for healthy child or her actual developing baby. There is also anticipated loss intertwined with the future loss of the baby and her brother.

REFERENCES

Austin, J., A. Semaka, and Hadjipavlou. G. 2014. "Conceptualizing Genetic Counseling as Psychotherapy in the Era of Genomic Medicine." *Journal of Genetic Counseling* 23: 903–909. https://doi.org/10.1007/s10897-014-9728-1.

Berg, Insoo Kim. 1994. *Family-Based Services: A Solution-Focused Approach*. New York: Norton.

Bernhardt, B. A., B. B. Biesecker, and C. L. Mastromarino. 2000. "Goals, Benefits, and Outcomes of Genetic Counseling: Client and Genetic Counselor Assessment." *American Journal of Medical Genetics* 94, no. 3: 189–97. http://www.ncbi.nlm.nih.gov/pubmed/10995504.

Biesecker, Barbara, Jehannine Austin, and Colleen Caleshu. 2017a. "Response to a Different Vantage Point Commentary: Psychotherapeutic Genetic Counseling, Is It?" *Journal of Genetic Counseling* 26, no. 2: 334–36. https://doi.org/10.1007/s10897-016-0025-z.

Biesecker, Barbara, Jehannine Austin, and Colleen Caleshu. 2017b. "Theories for Psychotherapeutic Genetic Counseling: Fuzzy Trace Theory and Cognitive Behavior Theory." *Journal of Genetic Counseling* 26, no. 2: 322–30. https://doi.org/10.1007/s10897-016-0023-1.

Cameron, L. D., Barbara Biesecker, E. Peters, J. M. Taber, and W. M. P. Klein. 2017. "Self-Regulation Principles Underlying Risk Perception and Decision Making within the Context of Genomic Testing." *Social and Personality Psychology Compass* 11, no. 5: e12315. https://doi.org/doi:10.1111/spc3.12315.

Corsini, Raymond. 1989. *Current Psychotherapies*. 4th ed. F. E. Peacock Publishers, Itasca.

Daly, M., J. Farmer, C. Harrop-Stein, S. Montgomery, M. Itzen, and J. W. Costalas. 1999. "Exploring Family Relationships in Cancer Risk Counseling Using the Genogram." *Cancer Epidemiology, Biomarkers and Prevention* 8, 4(Pt 2): 393–98.

Ellis, Albert. 1957. "Rational Psychotherapy and Individual Psychology." *Journal of Individual Psychology* 13: 38–44.

Eunpu, Deborah L. 1997. "Systemically-Based Psychotherapeutic Techniques in Genetic Counseling." *Journal of Genetic Counseling* 6, no. 1: 1–20. https://doi.org/10.1023/A:1025630917735.

France, Kenneth. 2014. *Crisis Intervention: A Handbook of Immediate Person-to-Person Help*. 6th ed. Springfield Illinois: Charles C. Thomas Pub. Ltd.

Gilligan, Carol. 1989. *Mapping the Moral Domain: A Contribution of Women's Thinking to Psychological Theory and Education*. Cambridge, MA: Harvard University Press.

Hunsley, John, and Gina Di Guilio. 2002. "Dodo Bird, Phoenix, or Urban Legend? The Question of Psychotherapy Equivalence." *Scientific Review of Mental Health Practice* 1, no. 1: 11–22.

Kessler, Seymour. 1979. *Genetic Counseling: Psychological Dimensions*. New York: Academic Press.

Kessler, Seymour. 1984. "Psychological Aspects of Genetic Counseling. III. Management of Guilt and Shame." *American Journal of Medical Genetics* 17: 673–97. https://doi.org/10.1002/ajmg.1320170320.

Kessler, Seymour. 1997. "Psychological Aspects of Genetic Counseling. IX. Teaching and Counseling." *Journal of Genetic Counseling* 6, no. 3: 287–95. https://doi.org/10.1023/A:1025676205440.

Knekt, P., E. Heinonen, K. Härkäpää, A. Järvikoski, E. Virtala, J. Rissanen, O. Lindfors, and Helsinki Psychotherapy Study Group. 2015. "Randomized Trial on the Effectiveness of Long- and Short-Term Psychotherapy on Psychosocial Functioning and Quality of Life during a 5-Year Follow-Up." *Psychiatry Research* 229, no. 1–2: 381–88. https://doi.org/10.1016/j.psychres.2015.05.113.

Knekt, P., E. Virtala, T. Härkänen, M. Vaarama, J. Lehtonen, and O. Lindfors. 2016. "The Outcome of Short- and Long-Term Psychotherapy 10 Years after Start of Treatment." *Psychological Medicine* 46, no. 6: 1175–88. https://doi.org/10.1017/S0033291715002718.

Koocher, Gerald P., Erin K. Curtiss, and Krista E. Patton. 2001. "Medical Crisis Counseling in a Health Maintenance Organization: Preventive Intervention." *Professional Psychology Research and Practice* 32, no. 1: 52–8. https://doi.org/DOI: 10.1037/0735-7028.32.1.52.

Lazarus, R. S., and S. Folkman. 1984. *Stress, Appraisal, and Coping. Behaviour Research and Therapy.* New York: Springer Publishing Company.

Lieberman, M. A., and Irvin Yalom. 1992. "Brief Group Psychotherapy for the Spousally Bereaved: A Controlled Study." *International Journal of Group Psychotherapy* 42, no. 1: 117–32.

Lipinski, Shawn E., Michael J. Lipinski, Leslie G. Biesecker, and Barbara B. Biesecker. 2006. "Uncertainty and Perceived Personal Control among Parents of Children with Rare Chromosome Conditions: The Role of Genetic Counseling." *American Journal of Medical Genetics Part C: Seminars in Medical Genetics* 142C, no. 4: 232–40. https://doi.org/10.1002/ajmg.c.30107.

Luborsky, L., B. Singer, and L. Luborsky. 1976. "Comparative Studies of Psychotherapies: Is It True That 'Everybody Has Won and All Must Have Prizes'?" *Proceedings of the Annual Meeting of the American Psychopathology Association* 64: 3–22.

Miller, Jean Baker. 1976. *Toward a New Psychology of Women.* Boston: Beacon Press.

Parkes, Colin Murray, and Holly G. Prigerson. 2010. *Bereavement: Studies of Grief in Adult Life.* 2nd ed. New York: Routledge.

Peters, June A., Lindsey Hoskins, Sheila Prindiville, Regina Kenen, and Mark H. Greene. 2006. "Evolution of the Colored Eco-Genetic Relationship Map (CEGRM) for Assessing Social Functioning in Women in Hereditary Breast-Ovarian (HBOC) Families." *Journal of Genetic Counseling* 15, no. 6: 477–89. https://doi.org/10.1007/s10897-006-9042-7.

Rogers, Carl. 1951. *Client-Centered Therapy: Its Current Practice, Implications and Theory.* London: Constable.

Rogers, Carol. 1980. *A Way of Being.* New York: Houghton Mifflin.

Rosenthal, E., Leslie G. Biesecker, and Barbara B. Biesecker. 2001. "Parental Attitudes toward a Diagnosis in Children with Unidentified Multiple Congenital Anomaly Syndromes." *American Journal of Medical Genetics* 103, no. 2: 106–14.

Shazer, Steve de. 1985. *Keys to Solution in Brief Therapy.* New York: W. W. Norton & Company.

Smith, Elsie J. 2006. "The Strength-Based Counseling Model." *Counseling Psychologist* 34, no. 13: 13–79. https://doi.org/10.1177/0011000005277018.

Stern, Alexandra Minna. 2012. *Telling Genes: The Story of Genetic Counseling in America.* Baltimore: Johns Hopkins University Press.

Wampold, Bruce. 2001. *The Great Psychotherapy Debate: Models, Methods, and Findings.* New York: Routledge.

Weil, John. 2000. *Psychosocial Genetic Counseling.* New York: Oxford University Press.

Worden, J. William. 2009. *Grief Counseling and Grief Therapy: A Handbook for the Mental Health Practitioner.* 4th ed. New York: Springer Publishing Company.

Yalom, Irvin. 2005. *Theory and Practice of Group Psychotherapy.* 5th ed. New York: Basic Books.

CHAPTER 10

Research in Genetic Counseling

Genetic counselors have been participating in research for decades. Historically, patients were primarily evaluated in academic medical centers where research into the origins and natural history of rare disease occurred. Within these studies of genetic conditions counselors often consented participants, managed protocols, provided clinical counseling, wrote institutional review board protocols, and contributed to study implementation, data analysis, and publication. Such opportunities have facilitated counselors' development of clinical research skills at the intersection of the counseling and research enterprises.

From this origin in rare disease research, genetic counselors have advanced their research participation to include government-funded research in clinical genomics, undiagnosed disease, and laboratory studies on the penetrance of gene variants and subsequent disease risk. The era of precision medicine offers further opportunities for genetic counselors to participate in research addressing the clinical translation of sequencing technologies (Biesecker 2018). Genetic counselors working alongside social and behavioral scientists, including investigators with training in health psychology, social psychology, and public health, are generating valuable evidence. For example, within the National Institutes of Health's Clinical Sequencing Evidence-Generating Research (CSER) consortia, genetic counselors were team members on a multisite effort to follow recipients of medically actionable secondary findings. Through this collaboration, genetic counselors returned the secondary findings, made follow-up recommendations to patients, collated findings across studies, interviewed participants to assess the outcomes of receiving this information, and led the writing of the manuscript for publication (Hart et al. 2018). This effort

> **Text Box 10.1**
>
> 1. Find researchers with similar interests.
> 2. Ask if you can join their research meetings.
> 3. Absorb the research language and culture.
> 4. Keenly observe how the team works.
> 5. Take notes on your relevant clinical insights.
> 6. Contribute those insights to the team.

exemplifies the significant contribution genetic counselors can make to the design and execution of team science. Published results from return of secondary findings revealed no evidence of psychological distress but limited communication of risks to first-degree relatives (Hart et al. 2018). As clinicians on the forefront of genomics translation, it is often the counselors who are keenly aware of where evidence is needed to guide clinical care and who are in a position to use the evidence to change practice. In this case, the findings suggested the need for interventions to enhance communication with at-risk relatives and cascade testing.

Box 10.1 provides suggestions for how counselors can join a research team.

RESEARCH LED BY GENETIC COUNSELORS

For years genetic counselors have been publishing their studies in the *Journal of Genetic Counseling*. Many are thesis studies executed by graduate students. Increasingly, genetic counselors are leading the design, execution, and publication of larger studies. An example of a study designed by a genetic counselor is a trial that randomized clients at 25% and 50% risk of having a pathogenic *BRCA1* variant to receive a problem-based coping intervention versus patient-centered (usual care) genetic counseling (McInerney-Leo et al. 2004). As hypothesized based on prior evidence, clients randomized to the problem-based coping intervention had fewer depressive symptoms at follow-up than clients who underwent patient-centered counseling. Results suggest that cancer counseling that enhances problem-based coping may improve psychological well-being more effectively that usual care. This example illustrates the value of assessing practice interventions in trials, with the caveat that the findings need to be replicated in other studies.

Erby, Roter, and Biesecker (2011) designed and conducted a process study called the Genetic Counseling Video Project that used simulated prenatal and cancer genetics clients to capture common genetic counseling practices. They analyzed the communication using Roter Interaction Analysis System (RIAS)-coded dialogue from videotaped sessions that the participant counselors rated as very similar to their clinical practice (Roter and Larson 2002). In cancer genetics, the genetic counselor consistently dominated the session with information that was dense and technical and required higher literacy skills (Erby et al. 2011). This counselor-led study provided key evidence that counselors spend more time providing complicated information rather than interacting with clients to understand how they are processing their risk status (Roter and Larson 2002). This finding has been replicated in recent studies of genetic counseling (Joseph et al. 2018; Kelly et al. 2015). Communicating detailed genetic information seems to be the dominant practice model, even though it is unlikely to be effective with most clients, particularly those with lower scientific and health literacy and less formal education (Joseph et al. 2017, 2018).

Genetic counselor Marion McAllister conducted a study with the goal of identifying outcomes valued by clinical genetics patients (McAllister and Dearing 2015). Results were used to develop and validate the Genetic Counseling Outcome Scale (GCOS) in the United Kingdom. The importance of patient-reported outcomes is reflected in the widespread efforts to promote Patient-Reported Outcome (PRO) research in medicine (Deshpande et al. 2011). The evidence from these studies can be used to tailor genetic counseling according to what is most highly valued by patients, leading to a closer match between the counseling process and client outcomes.

RESEARCH AS A PRIORITY FOR THE PROFESSION

The National Society of Genetic Counselors (NSGC) has long recognized the importance of research in genetic counseling, as illustrated by selected paper presentations at its annual conference. As the society has grown and research evolved, multiple research sessions are offered at the conference. NSGC has a research special interest group and has established protocols for developing evidence-based practice guidelines (https://www.nsgc.org/p/cm/ld/fid=70). Further, NSGC appointed an outcomes task force, recognizing the need for established research and practice outcomes (https://www.nsgc.org/p/bl/ar/blogaid=253). One goal is to enhance opportunities for reimbursement of services, and another is to achieve standardization in client outcomes for research.

> **Text Box 10.2**
>
> 1. Ask "why?" in clinic and in the classroom.
> 2. Look up answers to your "why?" questions.
> 3. Take note when there is no answer.
> 4. Attend to what interests you most.
> 5. Find others with the same question.

The Accreditation Council for Genetic Counseling requires students to have opportunities to perform research within their training programs as a component of the group's accreditation (http://www.gceducation.org/Pages/Standards.aspx). In accordance with this training standard, genetic counseling graduate students are publishing increasingly rigorous thesis studies in peer-reviewed journals (Hooker et al. 2014; Schaa et al. 2015; Helwig et al. 2019). Box 10.2 provides suggestions on how to generate a novel research question.

NEED FOR EVIDENCE-BASED PRACTICE

As the profession has matured, there is an increasing need for evidence-based practice. Beyond endorsement of research as a priority by our professional society and accreditation body, leading voices among genetic counselors have acknowledged the critical need for evidence-based practice (McAllister and Dearing 2015). One notable indicator of a leap in the quality of research is the rising impact factor for the *Journal of Genetic Counseling*, which frequently publishes studies of genetic counseling conducted by genetic counselors. Well-designed studies can yield data to inform practice. Increasingly, genetic counselors have designed and executed experiments; for example, to assess labeling of uncertain genome sequencing results (Hellwig et al. 2018). Genetic counselors can use results from this study to make laboratory decisions about how to parse uncertainty in labeling variant results.

In addition to experimental studies, systematic reviews of the literature are used to assess areas where there may be sufficient evidence to inform best clinical practices. For example, a systematic review of randomized controlled trials in genetic counseling yielded compelling evidence that telegenetic counseling is as effective or non-inferior to usual care in the cancer setting (Athens et al. 2017). The review identified fifty-four randomized controlled trials published over twenty-five years that assessed patient-related outcomes. Twenty-seven of these studies included an intervention arm hypothesized to enhance genetic counseling, and in many of them the data supported the hypothesis. Remarkably, the review identified consistency among assessment of the genetic counseling outcomes: psychological well-being, knowledge, decisional conflict/regret, and satisfaction. Yet these constructs differed in how they were defined and assessed across studies. Despite the consistency in assessing psychological well-being as a key outcome of genetic counseling, the variation in measurement precluded cross-study assessment of outcomes for meta-analyses.

While strides have been made in identifying outcomes of genetic counseling (McCuaig et al. 2018, Redlinger-Grosse K et al. 2016), to obtain evidence that can be used to inform practice, further alignment in selection of outcomes and how they are assessed is a research priority. Results from the literature review of clinical trials constitute an example of evidence that can be used to guide practice in the cancer setting. Generally, studies likely to have the greatest impact on informing practice effectiveness will be quantitative and have generalizable results. Research hierarchies rank systematic literature reviews with meta-analyses at the top of the quantitative list for impact. Compiling data from numerous studies and reassessing the data with a larger sample results in greater statistical power to arrive at evidence-based outcomes. These types of studies will be an important source of evidence to establish best practices in genetic counseling.

Experimental study designs also appear near the top of research hierarchies. Examples include randomized controlled trials where a counseling intervention may be compared to usual care. If such interventions are found to be promising, they can be disseminated into clinical settings for further assessment.

Qualitative methods often appeal to genetic counselors as they make use of our patient-related skills. For example, with some additional training counselors can conduct interviews, run focus groups, design open-ended questions for surveys, and lead community-based participatory research. Generally, these methods are exploratory and are used to describe a poorly understood phenomenon. As such, findings from qualitative research are often used to generate hypotheses that can be tested in subsequent research. Results can be important in stakeholder research in identifying perspectives that are likely to differ from those of clinicians or researchers. Because we as genetic counselors are seeking to understand how our clients perceive and respond to genetic conditions or risk, it is not surprising that we value information provided by our clients and other stakeholders. Exploratory findings can reveal previously unrecognized or unknown perspectives. Many studies of stakeholders, such as patients and families, are qualitative to minimize providers designing studies that are biased to reflect their perspective rather than that of our clients. Outcomes from exploratory research often is used to inform downstream quantitative studies where hypotheses are tested but is often insufficient to inform clinical practice.

RESEARCH TRAINING

Genetic counselors may elect to pursue a doctoral degree related to genetic counseling and conduct their dissertation research on a topic of direct or indirect relevance. While opportunities to conduct research do not necessitate higher education, those with doctoral-level training are better equipped to lead investigative teams and develop research programs. Genetic counselors with doctoral training may opt for positions that entail clinical and research responsibilities, such as implementing clinical trials of counseling interventions. Others may prefer one area over the other and contour their work accordingly.

In the United States, as of mid-2019, no doctoral programs in genetic counseling exist. It is arguable whether they are needed given the opportunities to earn degrees in health psychology, social psychology, health communication, health education, health services, bioethics, public policy, and other health-related specialties. Within each of these specialty areas there is scholarship that can be appropriated for genetic counseling research. For example, risk perception, its relation to worry and their interactive effects on health behaviors have been studied by health and social psychologists. These constructs are related to genetic information and how our clients respond to it.

A Ph.D. in genetic counseling may never be created given the broad range of research, the clinical nature of genetic counseling, and the lack of a singular circumscribed scholarship. Not having a Ph.D. that is specifically in genetic counseling is unlikely to be a detriment to individuals or to the profession as those who complete their doctoral training make contributions to the greater genetic counseling literature via their research publications irrespective of the degree that they earn. One could further argue that diversity of specialization in graduate studies and a breadth of published scholarship will broaden the research base for genetic counseling to inform practice.

You may wonder whether a genetic counselor interested in research should pursue doctoral training. As described, additional training is not required to make a valuable contribution in research teams. However, a counselor who is ambitious to focus her career on research alongside or instead of pursuing clinical care, would need to earn a doctorate to be successful as a researcher. One example of advanced training that may come to mind is genomics; some have taken this route, and others likely will do so in the future. These scholars are choosing to become geneticists as well as counselors rather than advancing their training in genetic counseling research per se. It represents an effort to broaden one's expertise into laboratory genetics rather than pursue research that advances understanding of clients' responses to genomic information to inform genetic counseling practice. Interestingly, some investigators with a Ph.D. in genomics opt for additional training in genetic counseling. All are laudable pursuits that contribute to the advancement of science, but these professionals will end up with different areas of expertise. For example, doctoral-level research by genetic counselors in social and behavioral research aims to further the scope of research in the clinical translation of genomics and genetic counseling. Investigators with expertise in genomics are more likely to pursue laboratory or epidemiology research.

Even without further training, many genetic counselors have identified opportunities to work in research teams. Often this happens, as introduced earlier, in rare disease research, because genetic counselors work in academic or research medical centers where research is often conducted. Counselors are often members of large research teams who recognize opportunities to partner with colleagues. Others may learn research skills through continuing education, and still others may be mentored by researchers and learn "on the job." Finding a research mentor can be a critical resource for research guidance. Research endeavors can be an interesting way to expand your expertise as a genetic counselor, and the rewards include furthering your professional relationships and collaborations, analyzing data and writing papers to submit for peer-review publication. These opportunities represent ways to make significant contributions to the field of genetic counseling as a researcher. Box 10.3 provides suggestions on how you can advance a research question.

Text Box 10.3

---

1. Find a research mentor (official or unofficial).
2. Determine whether your question is exploratory,
3. Or whether it is experimental.
4. Devour the literature on the topic.
5. Think about where your question fits in.
6. Work with your mentor to design a study.

KEY RESEARCH GAPS IN GENETIC COUNSELING

In 2017, the genetic counseling profession arrived at an historical juncture where the number of individuals receiving results from genomic testing and seeking genetic counseling, and the number of funded positions available, exceeded the number of genetic counselors available to fill them by hundreds. An NSGC workforce study reported that there would not be enough graduates from the US programs to fill these positions and that this trend was predicted to continue for years to come as precision medicine unfolds. (www.health.nsw.gov.au/workforce/alliedhealth/Documents/gsw-final-report.pdf). The previously mentioned literature review by Athens et al. (2017) included thirty-one studies that compared patient outcomes from an alternative delivery mode versus in-person genetic counseling. Alternative delivery modes included telephone counseling (Chang et al. 2016) and an electronic platform such as a CD-ROM or web-based platform (Green et al. 2001, 2005). The studies each found that the more cost-effective alternative service delivery mode was non-inferior or equivalent to usual in-person care as assessed by patient outcomes. These data support alternative delivery options that are efficient, lower in cost, and effective (Chang et al. 2016). Implementing these findings paves the way to the future of genetic counseling where evidence informs clinical practice. While this evidence addresses a service delivery mode rather than a counseling intervention, it represents an advancement in health services research in genetic counseling. Taken together, these studies may mark the first set of consistent findings from cost-effective low burden service delivery interventions shown to be as effective, or no worse than the more costly in-person usual care.

Data on the types of genetic results that may be communicated as effectively using online platforms provide another opportunity to inform ways to prioritize clients with significant health threats or personal loss for in-person care. One trial to assess return of carrier results to adults enrolled in a clinical genomic sequencing study found a web-based custom result platform to be non-inferior to in-person genetics education (counseling was offered separately) (Biesecker et al. 2018). These carrier results were of interest to participants to share with their adult children but represented no health risk, making them good candidates for a study of results via an alternative delivery mode because the risk of harm was low. Related research will continue to refine the ways that genomic information can be effectively delivered at a lower cost and burden to the client, while reserving in-person genetic counseling for more challenging cases that involve significant health threats, difficult patient decisions, and challenges faced by patients living with serious illness or disability. Novel interventions for assessment include the use of chatbots and other artificial intelligence interventions. Evidence for tiered service delivery modes can be used to maximize the time of expert genetic counselors for challenging cases and elevate the stature of the genetic counseling profession.

HEALTH BEHAVIOR AND SOCIAL PSYCHOLOGY THEORIES

Like the psychological counseling theories presented in Chapter 9 frame clinical practice, health behavior theories can be instrumental in framing genetic counseling research. Generally, social and behavioral research methods are most relevant to assessing outcomes from genetic counseling. They can be used to design studies to assess how clients perceive and use genomic information, and how well genetic counseling facilitates informed decision making. Even if you don't intend to pursue further training in research, becoming familiar with health behavior theories is an asset in reviewing research publications and in interpreting the results as they may relate to clinical care (Glanz et al. 2015).

Advanced training in health psychology often entails conducting research framed by behavior theory, such as follow-up use of health care following receipt of a test result indicating an elevated risk of cancer (Cameron et al. 2017). Theoretically framed research contributes to the evidence base for translational genomics and helps to broaden understanding of when and how individuals benefit from receipt of genetic information (Gray et al. 2017). Further, it links research in genetic counseling to published studies by the design parallels. Theoretically informed research significantly elevates the caliber of genetic counseling research and represents progress in genetic counseling research as it seeks to answer some of the most pressing questions facing the clinical translation of genomics.

Much of social and behavioral research is framed by health behavior and social psychology theories that are well established in the scientific literature and supported by evidence. The majority of these theories describe the thinking, feeling, and behavior of adults related to a health risk or condition and are referred to as interpersonal theories. Use of relevant theories facilitates selection of variables that have been conceptually posited to affect patient outcomes. Publications of health behavior research provide examples of studies framed by behavior theory that yield evidence of the role of factors that predict health decisions and their behavioral outcomes.

Three common intrapersonal health behavior theories are the Health Belief Model (HBM), the theories of reasoned action and planned behavior (TPB), and self-regulation theory. Each of these theories has been used to frame studies of decisions to receive genetic risk information (Cameron et al. 2017; Gooding et al. 2006). The HBM posits that individuals' perceptions of susceptibility, severity, benefits, and barriers are core constructs in predicting behaviors to avoid a negative health outcome. The model includes the modifying factors of knowledge, character traits, socioeconomic variables, cues to action (activation of readiness), and self-efficacy (confidence in one's ability to take action). Most often the HBM has been used to promote uptake of recommended health behaviors such as screening and prevention. Examples of prominent studies framed by the HBM are colonoscopy and mammography screening (Murphy et al. 2014; Williams, Wilkerson, and Holt 2018). In the genetics literature, studies of HBM have been used to frame decisions to undergo testing or use results from genetic testing to reduce one's health risk (Cyr, Dunnagan, and Haynes 2010; Horne et al. 2018; Sagi, Shiloh, and Cohen 1992).

The theory of reasoned action and the related theory of planned behavior have the following as their core theoretical constructs: attitudes (toward the risk or condition), subjective norms (normative values/expectations), perceived personal control (one's ability to influence the risk), intentions, and behavioral outcomes. A number of modifying variables have been studied, including risk perception and perceptions of uncertainty (Wade et al. 2012). In the genetics literature, studies framed by the theory of planned behavior include return of results studies in genomics and assessment of intentions to undergo prenatal testing and to enroll in treatment protocols (Gooding et al. 2006; Lakeman et al. 2009; Seaborn et al. 2016; Wolff et al. 2011).

The theory of self-regulation represents cyclical self-control and has the following as its core constructs: appraisals (of the health threat), health-related beliefs (about the disease or recommended action), timeline, consequences, and self-relevant beliefs. It also encompasses susceptibility to control, representation of the self, and strategies for self-protection. Self-regulation theory has been used most extensively in understanding how perceived threat influences downstream health-related decisions and behaviors. Leventhal and colleagues used concepts from self-regulation theory to create the Common Sense Model of Self-Regulation that has been promoted for its relevance in genetics studies (Cameron et al. 2017; Gooding et al. 2006). The core constructs of this model are perceptions of identity, cause, timeline, consequences, and controllability. Patients' perceptions of these characteristics of their illness or inherited risk determine how great a threat they perceive the condition is and how well they can manage that threat.

Related to these commonly used theories is the transactional theory of stress and coping, which describes a person's response to a health threat and involves primary and secondary appraisals of the threat, coping efficacy, and adaptation to the threat. Lazarus and Folkman's theory has been used in studies of a number of health threats (1984), such as a cancer diagnosis. In genetics, it has most often been applied to coping with uncertainty in unknown or rare diagnoses (Bell et al. 2019; Truitt et al. 2012; Yanes et al. 2017). The perceived threat of the condition and/or its uncertainty is manifested as stress. As most people respond to stressful events, patients and parents of patients appraise the threat to determine ways that it may best be managed. Initial appraisals work to construct meaning from the threat, in terms of the child's life and the family's life, as well as existential meaning.

From there parents and patients engage in secondary appraisals that involve conducting an inventory of their resources. These include assessing their level of confidence that they can persevere, finding ways to have some control over the situation, and reviewing their success in managing past stressors. Secondary appraisals precede and inform coping strategies that are accessible and may help parents manage the stress. There are many that are categorized as problem-focused and emotion-focused. Problem- or task-focused coping involves taking actions to address the stress—for example, working to find specialists to consult with (directed at the primary threat) and participating in an advocacy group (indirectly addressing the threat). There are coping strategies that are indirectly useful, such as sharing concerns with friends who can be counted on to respond in useful ways.

Emotion-focused coping addresses the stress from a health threat in the absence of tasks to be undertaken or when problem-focused coping is not useful. Emotion-focused coping serves to reduce the negative emotions of stress. Common examples are confiding one's fears to a trusted confidant, distracting oneself to avoid engaging in negative emotions, and reframing negative emotions into more hopeful ones.

When coping is more effective than not, over time parents and patients adapt to the health threat, although this is rarely a permanent state. New symptoms may arise, or a screening evaluation may reintroduce the health threat and the cycle of appraising, coping, and adapting begins anew. Most of us use healthy, effective coping strategies that allow us to adapt to the stress over time. This cycle of adapting leads to appraisals of our resources to manage it, inventorying what has been or may be successful, and choosing (consciously or subconsciously) ways to cope to reduce negative consequences of the stress. Maladaptive coping leads to ineffectual management of stressors by disruptions in the process of adapting.

Given the universality of the transactional theory of stress and coping in responding to stress, genetic counselors can relate this theory to their own lives and adopt it to frame their counseling practice in helping patients adapt to threatening genetic information. If, during counseling sessions, we keep in mind that early on patients and parents are simply trying to assess what has happened and give it meaning, we will recognize that the timing is not yet right for addressing secondary appraisals or coping. The process takes time, and as patients and parents come to find meaning, they are able to move forward to assess their resources and brainstorm coping strategies to help them manage. One study that randomized clients at significant risk for having a *BRCA1* variant to receive a problem-solving intervention aimed at identifying potential coping strategies or usual client-centered care found that the problem-solving intervention based on the transactional theory of stress and coping led to fewer depressive symptoms at follow-up (McInerney-Leo et al. 2004).

Interpersonal models are used to assess health behaviors among groups of people. Social cognitive theory assesses a number of constructs that consider the environment and situation. Core constructs include behavioral capacity, expectations, self-control, observational learning, reinforcements, self-efficacy, emotional coping responses, and reciprocal determination. Social cognitive theory can be used to assess environmental influences on the use of genetic information, a topic largely unaddressed in the research literature. Influences may include the shared experience of risk within extended families. Related questions pertain to how genomics may be offered within a fractionated health care delivery system where patients struggle to obtain routine care, much less have access to specialty follow-up care. Studies of the process of offering new technologies, such as genome sequencing, can be assessed and used to inform how services are designed and implemented to successfully reach patients.

RESEARCH IN GENETIC COUNSELING AND TRANSLATIONAL GENOMICS

Some of the research questions of greatest importance to the field of genetic counseling at the time this text was written originate from the translation of genomic sequencing into clinical care. Critical research questions include how to most efficiently and effectively consent clients to genome sequencing; strategies to manage clients' expectations of results; evidence-based best practices in return of uncertain results and secondary findings; and interventions assessed to facilitate and streamline medically actionable results return and appropriate follow-up care. It's also important to assess the overt and implicit processes that patients experience in anticipation and receipt of genomic information that can affect its usefulness in managing health threats and pursuit of health care and notification of at-risk relatives. Also needed are strategies for genetic counselors to partner effectively with clients from more diverse backgrounds who may have low scientific and health literacy.

As called for by the *All of Us* research program, scalable approaches to return of results will be needed when large swaths of the population undergo sequencing. Discerning when clinical outcomes for participants derive from in-person genetic counseling will continue to be important to assess. Experimental trials will be important in comparing delivery modes. This wealth of research questions represents an exciting opportunity for genetic counselors to conduct social and behavioral studies in the translation of genomics. We can be at the forefront of this evolution in genomics by collaborating with social and behavioral scientists and by pursuing training to become lead investigators (Turbitt and Biesecker 2019).

SUMMARY

Genetic counselors are likely to continue to expand in their active participation in research as genomics becomes integrated into mainstream medicine and novel research opportunities emerge. Those practicing in a research environment are well situated to design clinical experiments to address a number of the research questions related to translation of genomics. Collectively for the profession, generation of evidence will enhance practice so that patient-reported outcomes demonstrate we are effectively meeting our clients' needs.

REFERENCES

Athens, Barbara A., Samantha L. Caldwell, Kendall L. Umstead, Philip D. Connors, Ethan Brenna, and Barbara B. Biesecker. 2017. "A Systematic Review of Randomized Controlled Trials to Assess Outcomes of Genetic Counseling." *Journal of Genetic Counseling* 26, no. 5: 902–33. https://doi.org/10.1007/s10897-017-0082-y.

Bell, M., B. B. Biesecker, J. Bodurtha, and H. L. Peay. 2019. "Uncertainty, Hope, and Coping Efficacy among Mothers of Children with Duchenne/Becker Muscular Dystrophy." *Clinical Genetics* [Epub before print]. https://doi.org/10.1111/cge.13528.

Biesecker, B. B. 2018. "Genetic Counselors as Social and Behavioral Scientists in the Era of Precision Medicine." *American Journal of Medical Genetics C: Seminars in Medical Genetics* 178, no. 1: 10–14. https://doi.org/10.1002/ajmg.c.31609.

Biesecker, B. B., K. L. Lewis, K. L. Umstead, J. J. Johnston, E. Turbitt, K. P. Fishler, . . . L. G. Biesecker. 2018. "Web Platform vs In-Person Genetic Counselor for Return of Carrier Results from Exome Sequencing: A Randomized Clinical Trial." *JAMA Internal Medicine* 178, no. 3: 338–46. https://doi.org/10.1001/jamainternmed.2017.8049.

Cameron, L. D., Barbara Biesecker, E. Peters, J. M. Taber, and W. M. P. Klein. 2017. "Self-Regulation Principles Underlying Risk Perception and Decision Making within the Context of Genomic Testing." *Social and Personality Psychology Compass* 11, no. 5: e12315. https://doi.org/doi:10.1111/spc3.12315.

Chang, Y., A. M. Near, K. M. Butler, A. Hoeffken, S. L. Edwards, A. M. Stroup, . . . J. S. Mandelblatt. 2016. "Economic Evaluation alongside a Clinical Trial of Telephone versus In-Person Genetic Counseling for BRCA1/2 Mutations in Geographically Underserved Areas." *Journal of Oncology Practice* 12, no. 1: e1–e13. https://doi.org/10.1200/JOP.2015.004838.

Cyr, A., T. A. Dunnagan, and G. Haynes. 2010. "Efficacy of the Health Belief Model for Predicting Intention to Pursue Genetic Testing for Colorectal Cancer." *Journal of Genetic Counseling* 19, no. 2: 174–86. https://doi.org/10.1007/s10897-009-9271-7.

Deshpande, P. R., S. Rajan, B. L. Sudeepthi, and C. P. Abdul Nazir. 2011. "Patient-Reported Outcomes: A New Era in Clinical Research." *Perspectives in Clinical Research* 2, no. 4: 137–44. https://doi.org/10.4103/2229-3485.86879.

Erby, L. A., D. L. Roter, and B. B. Biesecker. 2011. "Examination of Standardized Patient Performance: Accuracy and Consistency of Six Standardized Patients over Time." *Patient Education and Counseling* 85, no. 2: 194–200. https://doi.org/10.1016/j.pec.2010.10.005.

Glanz, K., B. K. Rimer, and K. V. Viswanath. 2015. *Health Behavior and Health Education: Theory and Practice*. Fifth Edition. Jossey-Bass: San Francisco CA.

Gooding, H. C., K. Organista, J. Burack, and B. B. Biesecker. 2006. "Genetic Susceptibility Testing from a Stress and Coping Perspective." *Social Science and Medicine* 62, no. 8: 1880–890. https://doi.org/10.1016/j.socscimed.2005.08.041.

Gray, Stacy W., Sarah E. Gollust, Deanna Alexis Carere, Clara A. Chen, Angel Cronin, Sarah S. Kalia, . . . Robert C. Green. 2017. "Personal Genomic Testing for Cancer Risk: Results from the Impact of Personal Genomics Study." *Journal of Clinical Oncology* 35, no. 6: 636–44. https://doi.org/10.1200/JCO.2016.67.1503.

Green, M. J., A. M. McInerney, B. B. Biesecker, and N. Fost. 2001. "Education about Genetic Testing for Breast Cancer Susceptibility: Patient Preferences for a Computer Program or Genetic Counselor." *American Journal of Medical Genetics* 103, no. 1: 24–31. http://www.ncbi.nlm.nih.gov/pubmed/11562930.

Green, M. J., S. K. Peterson, M. W. Baker, L. C. Friedman, G. R. Harper, W. S. Rubinstein, . . . D. T. Mauger. 2005. "Use of an Educational Computer Program before Genetic Counseling for Breast Cancer Susceptibility: Effects on Duration and Content of Counseling Sessions." *Genetics in Medicine* 7, no. 4: 221–29. https://doi.org/10.109701.GIM.0000159905.13125.86.

Hart, M. R., B. B. Biesecker, C. L. Blout, K. D. Christensen, L. M. Amendola, K. L. Bergstrom, . . . L. A. Hindorff. 2018. "Secondary Findings from Clinical Genomic Sequencing: Prevalence, Patient Perspectives, Family History Assessment, and Health-Care Costs from a Multisite Study." *Genetics in Medicine* [Epub before print]. https://doi.org/10.1038/s41436-018-0308-x.

Hellwig, L. D., B. B. Biesecker, K. L. Lewis, L. G. Biesecker, C. A. James, and W. M. P Klein. 2018. "Ability of Patients to Distinguish among Cardiac Genomic Variant Subclassifications." *Circulation: Genomic and Precision Medicine* 11, no. 6: e001975. https://doi.org/10.1161/CIRCGEN.117.001975.

Hooker, G. W., H. Peay, L. Erby, T. Bayless, B. B. Biesecker, and D. L. Roter. 2014. "Genetic Literacy and Patient Perceptions of IBD Testing Utility and Disease Control: A Randomized Vignette Study of Genetic Testing." *Inflammatory Bowel Disease* 20, no. 5: 901–908. https://doi.org/10.1097/MIB.0000000000000021.

Horne, J., J. Madill, C. O'Connor, J. Shelley, and J. Gilliland. 2018. "A Systematic Review of Genetic Testing and Lifestyle Behaviour Change: Are We Using High-Quality Genetic Interventions and Considering Behaviour Change Theory?" *Lifestyle Genomics* 11, no. 1: 49–63. https://doi.org/10.1159/000488086.

Joseph, Galen, Robin Lee, Rena J. Pasick, Claudia Guerra, Dean Schillinger, and Sara Rubin. 2018. "Effective Communication in the Era of Precision Medicine: A Pilot Intervention with Low Health Literacy Patients to Improve Genetic Counseling Communication." *European Journal of Medical Genetics* [Epub before print]. https://doi.org/10.1016/j.ejmg.2018.12.004.

Joseph, Galen, R. J. Pasick, D. Schillinger, J. Luce, C. Guerra, and J. K. Y. Cheng. 2017. "Information Mismatch: Cancer Risk Counseling with Diverse Underserved Patients." *Journal of Genetic Counseling* 26, no. 5: 1090–104. https://doi.org/10.1007/s10897-017-0089-4.

Kelly, K. M., L. Ellington, N. Schoenberg, T. Jackson, S. Dickinson, K. Porter, ... M. Andrykowski. 2015. "Genetic Counseling Content: How Does It Impact Health Behavior?" *Journal of Behavioral Medicine* 38, no. 5: 766–76. https://doi.org/10.1007/s10865-014-9613-2.

Lakeman, P., A. M. Plass, L. Henneman, P. D. Bezemer, M. C. Cornel, and L. P. ten Kate. 2009. "Preconceptional Ancestry-Based Carrier Couple Screening for Cystic Fibrosis and Haemoglobinopathies: What Determines the Intention to Participate or Not and Actual Participation?" *European Journal of Human Genetics* 17, no. 8: 999–1009. https://doi.org/10.1038/ejhg.2009.1.

Lazarus, R. S., and S. Folkman. 1984. *Stress, Appraisal, and Coping. Behaviour Research and Therapy*.

McAllister, M., and A. Dearing. 2015. "Patient Reported Outcomes and Patient Empowerment in Clinical Genetics Services." *Clinical Genetics* 88, no. 2: 114–21. https://doi.org/10.1111/cge.12520.

McCuaig, Jeanna M., Susan Randall Armel, Melanie Care, Alexandra Volenik, Raymond H. Kim, and Kelly A. Metcalfe. 2018. "Next-Generation Service Delivery: A Scoping Review of Patient Outcomes Associated with Alternative Models of Genetic Counseling and Genetic Testing for Hereditary Cancer." *Cancers* (Basel) 10, no.11: 435. doi:10.3390/cancers10110435

McInerney-Leo, A., B. B. Biesecker, D. W. Hadley, R. G. Kase, T. R. Giambarresi, E. Johnson, ... J. P. Struewing. 2004. "BRCA1/2 Testing in Hereditary Breast and Ovarian Cancer Families: Effectiveness of Problem-Solving Training as a Counseling Intervention." *American Journal of Medical Genetics, Part A* 130A, no. 3: 221–27. https://doi.org/10.1002/ajmg.a.30265.

Murphy, C. C., S. W. Vernon, P. M. Diamond, and J. A. Tiro. 2014. "Competitive Testing of Health Behavior Theories: How Do Benefits, Barriers, Subjective Norm, and Intention Influence Mammography Behavior?" *Annals of Behavioral Medicine* 47, no. 1: 120–29. https://doi.org/10.1007/s12160-013-9528-0.

Redlinger-Grosse, Krista, Patricia McCarthy Veach, Stephanie Cohen, Bonnie S. LeRoy, Ian M. MacFarlane, Heather Zierhut. 2016. "Defining Our Clinical Practice: The Identification of Genetic Counseling Outcomes Utilizing the Reciprocal Engagement Model." *Journal of Genetic Counseling* 25, no. 2: 239–257. doi:10.1007/s10897-015-9864-2

Roter, Debra L., and S. Larson. 2002. "The Roter Interaction Analysis System (RIAS): Utility and Flexibility for Analysis of Medical Interactions." *Patient Education and Counseling* 46, no. 4: 243–51.

Sagi, M., S. Shiloh, and T. Cohen. 1992. "Application of the Health Belief Model in a Study on Parents' Intentions to Utilize Prenatal Diagnosis of Cleft Lip and/or Palate." *American Journal of Medical Genetics* 44, no. 3: 326–33. https://doi.org/10.1002/ajmg.1320440312.

Schaa, K. L., D. L. Roter, B. B. Biesecker, L. A. Cooper, and L. H. Erby. 2015. "Genetic Counselors' Implicit Racial Attitudes and Their Relationship to Communication." *Health Psychology* 34, no. 2: 111–19. https://doi.org/10.1037/hea0000155.

Seaborn, C., S. Suther, T. Lee, G. E. Kiros, A. Becker, E. Campbell, and J. Collins-Robinson. 2016. "Utilizing Genomics through Family Health History with the Theory of Planned Behavior: Prediction of Type 2 Diabetes Risk Factors and Preventive Behavior in an African American Population in Florida." *Public Health Genomics* 19, no. 2: 69–80. https://doi.org/10.1159/000443471.

Truitt, M., B. B. Biesecker, G. Capone, T. Bailey, and L. Erby. 2012. "The Role of Hope in Adaptation to Uncertainty: The Experience of Caregivers of Children with Down Syndrome." *Patient Education and Counseling* 87, no. 2: 233–38. https://doi.org/10.1016/j.pec.2011.08.015.

Turbitt, E., and B. B. Biesecker. 2019. "A Primer in Genomics for Social and Behavioral Researchers." *Translational Behavioral Medicine* [Epub before print]. doi:10.1093/tbm/ibz018.

Wade, C. H., S. Shiloh, S. W. Woolford, J. S. Roberts, S. H. Alford, T. M. Marteau, and B. B. Biesecker. 2012. "Modelling Decisions to Undergo Genetic Testing for Susceptibility to Common Health Conditions: An Ancillary Study of the Multiplex Initiative." *Psychology & Health* 27, no. 4: 430–44. https://doi.org/10.1080/08870446.2011.586699.

Williams, R. M., T. Wilkerson, and C. L. Holt. 2018. "The Role of Perceived Benefits and Barriers in Colorectal Cancer Screening in Intervention Trials among African Americans." *Health Education Research* 33, no. 3: 205–17. https://doi.org/10.1093/her/cyy013.

Wolff, K., K. Nordin, W. Brun, G. Berglund, and G. Kvale. 2011. "Affective and Cognitive Attitudes, Uncertainty Avoidance and Intention to Obtain Genetic Testing: An Extension of the Theory of Planned Behaviour." *Psychology & Health* 26, no. 9: 1143–55. https://doi.org/10.1080/08870441003763253.

Yanes, T., L. Humphreys, A. McInerney-Leo, and B. B. Biesecker. 2017. "Factors Associated with Parental Adaptation to Children with an Undiagnosed Medical Condition." *Journal of Genetic Counseling* 26, no. 4: 829–40. https://doi.org/10.1007/s10897-016-0060-9.

CHAPTER 11

Genetic Counseling in the Genomic Era

PERSPECTIVE

The longstanding approach to counseling about genetic testing has been based largely on the model of nondirective pre-test counseling with follow-up counseling of those patients who elect to proceed with genetic testing (Kessler 2001; Weil et al. 2006). This model was a natural response to several historical, sociocultural, demographic, and economic factors (see Chapter 2 on the history of genetic counseling). But it is time to revisit the utility and practicality of this model and the role of genetic counselors in the era of genomic medicine (Biesecker 2018; Brett et al. 2018; Patch and Middleton 2018).

To be sure, not all genetic counseling focuses on genetic testing. Other skills in genetic counselors' scope of practice and daily activities in a clinical setting include ongoing advocacy and education; clinical insight; providing psychotherapeutic counseling; breaking a diagnosis to a family; and serving as a resource to other medical care providers, to name a few. It is reasonable that these activities will continue for the foreseeable future because they are still critical and require a combined skill set unmatched by most other care providers. Thus, even though genetic counseling is often conflated with genetic testing, genetic testing is just one aspect of genetic counseling. Complex genetic testing such as exome/genome sequencing can be a powerful diagnostic tool but still often does not establish a diagnosis or prognosis and can create uncertainty (Hayeems et al. 2016). Genetic counselors need to be prepared to help patients understand and adapt to that uncertainty.

The genetic counseling profession was born during the 1970s and the ethos of the nascent profession reflected the greater social milieus (See Chapter 2). Women were starting to gain some measure of control over their reproductive decisions with the widespread availability of safe, legal abortion and birth control, as well as more and better economic opportunities. The longstanding paternalistic medical model of doctors deciding what was best for patients was beginning to erode. Patients were taking a greater role in their medical care and decision making. Genetic counselors and their patients were approximate mirror images of each other: middle-class and upper-middle-class women who shared many of the same values.

Genetic testing was limited in the number of conditions that were amenable to diagnosis. Treatments and interventions were sparse. Thus, only a fairly narrow segment of the patient population ever had reason to come in contact with genetic counselors. In the era before the internet, information about even relatively common conditions like Down syndrome and cystic fibrosis was hard to come by. Genetic testing was expensive, insurance reimbursement was uncertain, and there were only a limited number of labs that undertook genetic testing.

In this context, the traditional genetic counseling model made sense. Genetic counselors became de facto gatekeepers of genetic medicine because no one else was equipped to do it, and they were in the right place at the right time to fill that role. There wasn't much competition and there wasn't much profit.

THE CHANGING WORLD OF GENETIC COUNSELING AND GENETIC TESTING

But this picture has changed considerably. There are now thousands of genetic tests offered by many labs, for which genetic testing has become their sole or a significant source of their profits. Increased competition and improved technology have lowered the costs. Multigene panels and exome/genome sequencing reduce the need for expensive sequential testing, imaging studies, and non-genetic lab tests. Panels also reduce the role of specialist knowledge in test selection because they typically include all the differential diagnoses for a given condition, and phenotype has proven to be only a modest predictor of genotype for many genetic disorders. Insurance coverage, while far from perfect, is no worse for genetic testing than other areas of medical care. Genetic testing and screening are now offered to nearly all pregnant women in the United States and many other Westernized countries. The patient population is larger and more diverse, a diversity poorly reflected in the genetic counseling workforce. Oncologists, neurologists, cardiologists, surgeons, and other medical specialists and generalists have incorporated genetic testing into their practice and increasingly order testing themselves without the filter of a genetic counselor. After doing internet searches, patients come to our offices sometimes more knowledgeable about genetic conditions than we are. And the increasing presence of various forms of direct-to-consumer genetic testing have the potential—for better or worse—to make it simple for almost anyone to order a genetic test (Ramos and Weissman 2018).

So, what is the role of genetic counselors and genetic counseling in this new world order?

Genetic counselors are now employed as clinicians, clinical managers, program directors, government employees, administrators, laboratory specialists who serve as clinical advisors and go-betweens with the clinical community, scientific information officers, product specialists, genetic test product developers, database curators, and sales specialists. They work in both indirect and direct patient care.

Those working in direct patient care may see a shift from providing pre-test and post-test counseling for some tests. Many veteran genetic counselors may find this shift regrettable because of their understanding of the complex emotional and familial implications of entering into the genetic testing pathway, which is inevitably more complicated in its ramifications than a "simple blood test." Genetic counselors viewed themselves as playing a vital role in helping patients work through these ramifications such that clients are adequately prepared to adapt to and utilize the results and to determine if they were even ready to undergo genetic testing to begin with. The ideal genetic counseling session was a blend of educational and counseling skills that helped patients become empowered, educated, and emotionally adapted. The psychological and social component is what transforms an educational process into an opportunity for patients to experience personal growth, better adapt to their situation, feel a greater sense of control over their lives, and experience overall higher satisfaction. But, like it or not, there is reason to believe this pre-test counseling role will diminish, though not necessarily disappear, as more non-genetics health care providers order genetic testing or patients take it on themselves via direct-to-consumer testing.

For decades, almost all genetic counseling patients have either been affected by a genetic disorder or faced an increased risk for themselves or their children to develop a specific disorder. However, with the increasing clinical utility of genetic testing in helping prevent or reduce the risk for common disorders such as cancer, the growing recognition that many genetic conditions occur among people with no obvious risk factors, consumer marketing that may sometimes overstate the clinical utility of some tests, and the decreasing costs of testing, more and more patients will be healthy, apparently average-risk people who undergo genetic testing in hopes of better establishing their health risks and improving the medical and emotional management of those risks. This may result in a different set of psychological and social effects than in patients who had familial or medical risk factors for genetic disease. Test results that indicate a high risk of a life-threatening condition, dropped out of the blue on a patient who was not anticipating them, might result in different set of psychological complexities that require different ways of enabling patient adaptation and psychological growth.

Whether the potential decline of pre-test genetic counseling is a good thing is open to debate. Genetics is complicated, both technically and emotionally. Many patients and care providers are often not fully aware of this complexity, and there is a tendency to view genetic testing as "just another blood test." This alone may make a stronger case for more pre-test genetic counseling. But there has been little research to demonstrate whether pre-test counseling by a genetic counselor consistently results in better patient outcomes than pre-test counseling by other health care providers or by a well-designed decision aid, although some data support the contention that genetic counselors are better at interpreting genetic test results and identifying appropriate tests and the appropriate patients for those tests. Most of the studies in the articles noted below focused on cancer genetic counseling, leaving a wide range of genetic counseling specialties understudied.

For example, one study found that breast cancer patients whose genetic test results showed a variant of uncertain significance were more likely to undergo bilateral mastectomy if a genetic counselor was not directly involved with their care (Kurian et al. 2017). On the other hand, a study of genetic counseling for Alzheimer disease risk found no significant differences between genetic counselors and physicians in terms of patient anxiety, depression, and test-related distress at twelve months after the intervention (Green et al. 2015). A systematic review of randomized controlled trials in genetic counseling found that genetic counseling enhanced some patient outcomes, such as psychological well-being, knowledge, perceived risk, and satisfaction; however, the fact that disparate scales were used in these studies limited the ability to compare findings across studies (Athens et al. 2017). Similarly, a systematic review of outcome studies in genetic counseling concluded that genetic counseling can lead to increased knowledge, perceived personal control, positive health behaviors, and improved risk perception as well as decreased anxiety, cancer-related worry, and decisional conflicts (Madlensky et al. 2017). One study of video-based genetic counseling of patients with ovarian cancer suggested that genetic testing uptake was greater in patients who viewed a condensed genetic counseling video versus the previous practice of referral to a genetic counselor (Watson et al. 2016).

To a large extent, the relative superiority of various forms and practitioners of genetic counseling depends on how one defines success. Is success measured by genetic test uptake? Adherence to recommended screening, surgical, or risk-reducing strategies? Patient satisfaction? Adaptation? Information recall? Anxiety reduction? Appropriate test interpretation? Cost savings? Reduced disease incidence, morbidity, and/or mortality? More family members being tested? Until such outcomes are widely agreed on and weighted for importance, any discussion about the relative merits of genetic counseling strategies are meaningless.

A task force convened by the National Society of Genetic Counselors has published standards for the reporting of genetic counseling interventions that should help to improve standardization and therefore comparison across studies (Hooker et al. 2017). But genetic counselors' views may be influenced by unconscious biases and motivated blindness (see the discussion of conflict of interest in Chapter 7) in assessing their own effectiveness. Evaluation of the success of genetic counseling and of the effectiveness of genetic counselors should also include input from other stakeholders—patients, referring physicians, health insurers, researchers, etc.

Perhaps the population with the most at stake with the loss of pre-test genetic counseling are people with disabilities, their families, and their supporters. Although this population has criticized the prenatal diagnosis paradigm of screening for—and selecting out—fetuses with genetic conditions, it is also true that, paradoxically, genetic counselors are often the strongest supporters of this same population. Pre-test genetic counseling by a genetic counselor involves exploring the emotional, medical, and familial impact of genetic conditions and providing a careful explanation of what patients are signing up for when they enter the prenatal screening cascade. In the absence of this service, there is justifiable concern that prenatal screening for genetic and congenital disorders will become further routinized along with the many other tests of pregnancy—rubella titers, glucose levels, blood type, etc.—absent the soul-searching that prenatal screening should entail. Patients may be given pamphlets with an outline of prenatal screening and a brief discussion, which can get lost along with all of the other information typically provided by care providers during early pregnancy.

One study that recorded first prenatal visits of 210 patients with forty-five obstetrical providers found that less than 2% of the conversations included all the topics recommended by the American College of Obstetricians and Gynecologists. The discussion about fetal aneuploidy screening took place in 90% of visits. However, the discussions lasted on average less than two minutes. Only about half of the conversations mentioned that aneuploidy testing was a screen rather than a diagnostic test and just under 50% included mention that aneuploidy screening was a choice (Colicchia et al. 2016). A study in which twenty-one obstetricians were interviewed about aneuploidy screening found that most providers felt they had inadequate time to educate and counsel their patients (Gammon et al. 2016). Given the complexity of fetal aneuploidy screening, group or other alternative counseling strategies may be more beneficial for patients than relying on obstetric providers (Knutzen et al. 2013).

Whatever their role in ordering and/or interpreting genetic testing, what should remain key to clinical genetic counselors' role is perhaps the most critical part: enhancing psychological and social outcomes for patients. Better knowledge, reduced anxiety, and some other older measures of the outcomes of genetic counseling are at best poor predictors of the success of genetic counseling and patient satisfaction. Patients need to be psychologically enriched by the genetic counseling experience, and education is only one component of that enrichment and one that may not be relevant for some patients. Thus, while the potential diminution of pre-test genetic counseling is to be lamented, new ways of doing things does not spell the end of the world for the genetic counseling profession. Instead, it can open up new opportunities for genetic counselors to apply their skills and strengths.

Genetic counselors working in non-direct patient contact positions, such as in testing laboratories, are playing a greater role in clinical interpretation of test results, test development, educational support for clinical genetic counselors and non-genetics providers, and working with clinical counselors to help integrate test results into patient care. These duties require hands-on clinical knowledge, a good grasp of the psychological and social implications of test interpretation for the patient, and utilization of their own counseling skills in interacting with the medical community. Laboratory genetic counselors can play a key role in the delivery of genetic counseling services even if they do not interact directly with patients.

THE UTILITY OF THE CURRENT DEFINITION OF GENETIC COUNSELING

All of which begs the question: Does the current definition of genetic counseling adequately reflect the work of genetic counselors in the genomic era? The definition of genetic counseling was discussed in Chapter 3. Let's examine the definition again line by line to see how it may or may not fit into the clinical genomic landscape.

Genetic counseling is the process of helping people understand and adapt to the medical, psychological, and familial implications of genetic contributions to disease. This sentence implies a one-on-one interaction between a genetic counselor and a client/family, either in person or via e-connection, or possibly an interaction between one counselor and a smallish group. But as genetic information and test interpretation grows ever more complex, a session of roughly thirty to sixty minutes may be inadequate, inefficient, and ineffective in many situations. "Helping people understand" will become harder and harder. The clinical genetics clinic encounter usually involved a detailed physical examination and perhaps imaging and other ancillary studies to help limit the number of suspected diagnoses and targeted genetic tests. This was in part driven by costs—until recently, genetic testing was expensive, and obtaining insurance coverage could be a struggle. Now often it is economically and clinically more effective to order multiplex genetic tests that scan for large numbers of relevant genetic conditions. And it is likely that more and more people will undergo genetic testing without having first met with a genetic counselor, while it seems unlikely that most non-genetic professionals who order genetic testing for their patients will have spent adequate time and resources preparing patients for the limits, utility, advantages, and disadvantages of genetic testing. This holds true broadly across all clinical specialties—pediatrics, reproductive and prenatal clinics, neurology, cardiology, and oncology.

Several strategies for how to offer multiplex genetic testing or exome analysis have been proposed. These strategies break down test panels into broad categories and patients can opt to receive full or partial results depending on their preferences and on professional guidelines. But as genetic testing becomes increasingly integrated into routine clinical care, the tendency, especially for non-genetics clinicians, may be to simply say to patients, "We are going to test you for a bunch of genetic conditions and we will let you know if we turn up anything significant" and maybe provide a pamphlet or website for patients who want more specific information.

Once test results are available, especially those that yield ambiguous results or a result about a condition that the patient and/or provider was not expecting, patients may seek genetic counseling *after* they have undergone genetic testing. Thus, as noted above, genetic counseling may shift its focus from a service provided both before and after genetic testing to a service provided primarily after genetic testing. This would represent a dramatic paradigm shift for genetic counselors. The aspect of genetic counseling that explored the medical, personal, and psychological factors surrounding whether to undergo genetic testing and which test to have could fade into the background since many patients will have had their test ordered by a non-genetics specialist.

However, the other parts of the definition may still hold true. That is, the test results will still need to be interpreted in light of patients' family and medical histories. Education and counseling around decision making may then shift to what options are best for a patient, such as high-risk cancer screening, risk-reducing surgery, etc., rather than on the decision of whether to undergo genetic testing. Exploring the psychological impact of the test result can help families/patients adapt to their new risk status or diagnosis.

There is a potential concern, though, that genetic counseling could become mostly a matter of technical explanations to patients about their complicated test results and would lose the rich psychological and social component. Genetic counselors may come to be viewed as medical specialists who provide expertise on technical knowledge, and the counseling component could fade from the patient interaction. It would be a step backwards to the now largely defunct and ineffective educational model of genetic counseling.

SERVICE DELIVERY MODELS

What will need to continue to adapt, evolve, and expand are the service delivery models of genetic counseling and the way that technology is incorporate into patient care (Gordon et al. 2018; Stoll et al. 2018). If the predicted growth of genomic medicine is actually achieved, the one-on-one in-person genetic counseling session that relies almost entirely on the genetic counselor as the expert provider will likely be inadequate to meet the demands of providing service to the tens of millions of patients considering or undergoing increasingly complex and wide-ranging genetic tests. And, as noted above, the service may also wind up being geared primarily to post-test genetic counseling of patients who underwent testing through their own care providers or through direct-to-consumer services, rather than pre-test counseling based on specific risk factors and psychological and social exploration of the implications of genetic testing followed by post-test counseling by the same genetic counselor.

Some studies have found that patients are quite comfortable with, and may even prefer, receiving genomic results and interpretations online or through mobile phone apps (Biesecker et al. 2018). Patients may then seek genetic counseling to clarify what the results mean for them individually and how they might impact their health care and lifestyle. However, counselees typically wish to have a greater voice in setting the agenda for the session and may see genetic counseling as one source of advice and information, along with online resources, social media, support groups, primary care providers, and other medical specialists (Sweet et al. 2016).

One study found that website-based information about prenatally diagnosed diaphragmatic hernia helped improve expectant mothers' understanding of management strategies and maternal risks (Engels et al. 2013). Indeed, many genetic counselors are already supplementing in-person counseling with other service delivery models, such as telephone counseling, telegenetics, and group counseling (Cohen et al. 2013). Other providers are experimenting with a YouTube clinical genetics channel to provide educational resources for patients (Jones et al. 2016). Web-based tutoring systems may be effective in educating patients and helping them make decisions about genetic testing (Wolfe et al. 2015). Some privately owned companies offer web-based and/or telephonic genetic counseling exclusively.

Nonetheless, a substantial number of patients do not have familiarity and comfort with internet resources. Many lower socioeconomic groups have limited internet access. These issues are further compounded for non-English-speaking migrants and refugees. It is therefore critical that service delivery models provide new and creative ways to effectively and fairly deliver genetic counseling services to these generally underserved populations with lower health literacy (Joseph et al. 2017; Mette et al. 2016; Peterson et al. 2018; Woodson et al. 2015).

WHICH RESULTS SHOULD BE SHARED WITH PATIENTS?

Multigene panels or exome/genome sequencing studies typically cover a wide range of conditions, often including conditions for which the patient was not at apparent risk. This begs the question: "Which results should be shared with patients?"

The superficial answer is "All of them." After all, patients have a right to know all of the information that they or their insurer paid for. Patients own their test results, not the medical community. On the other hand, multigene panels, microarray testing, genome-wide association screens, and exome/genome sequencing can yield hundreds or thousands of results, not all of which can realistically and effectively be communicated to the patient. Patients should always have access to all of their test results, but what needs to be determined are which results are particularly important to patients at this point in their lives; these should be the primary focus of the genetic counseling session.

Because of the wide-ranging nature of these tests, many patients may have greater interests in some results than others. But clients who undergo a exome screen to search for a specific type of diagnosis, say a neurogenetic disorder, may also wish to be informed of their cancer risks or carrier status of recessive disorders to inform reproductive decisions. It is also possible that the patient did not meet with a genetic counselor prior to testing and may not have been fully prepared for the discovery of conditions unrelated to the primary reason that the testing was ordered to begin with. At the other end of the spectrum are healthy patients with no particular risk factors who underwent genetic testing with the somewhat unfocused desire to find out what health risks they may face during their lifetime and entered the testing pathway expecting to learn information about risks for a large number of unrelated common health conditions—cancer, dementia, diabetes, cardiovascular disease, etc.

The patient's expectations should be clarified upfront. The patient should be given the opportunity to set the direction and focus of the genetic counseling session. Open-ended questions along the lines of "What brings you to my office today?" and "What would you like to achieve during this appointment together?" give patients the opportunity to express their needs and desires. This process may involve some clarification and setting of realistic expectations on the part of the genetic counselor, particularly if the patient responds, "I want to know everything about all my test results." Especially with genome-wide association studies or exome/genome sequencing, genetic counselors should identify the broad range of conditions tested for and explain that a single genetic counseling session, from a practical standpoint, can cover only a portion of those results. In some cases, patients may be better served by scheduling multiple genetic counseling sessions in the immediate future or in the more distant future as the risk of different genetic diseases has greater salience.

A more complicated situation arises when patients state that they made the genetic counseling appointment because "My doctor told me to. I am not really sure why I am here." This may be genuinely true for some patients, but by and large most patients have a rough idea of why they are in our offices. However, they might be reluctant to acknowledge the reason, especially if it is about a sensitive subject, such as addressing the health condition that a parent or close sibling may have died from or some other topic that evokes a deep emotional reaction from the patient. Eliciting helpful responses from patients requires good counseling and interviewing skills. You might ask what conversations the patient had with the primary care provider or specialist that led to the recommendation to see a genetic counselor, and then ask how the patient felt or thought about the provider's recommendation. The genetic counselor could indicate what types of issues are discussed in a genetic counseling session and ask the patient which, if any, of those issues might be of particular interest or importance at this point in the patient's life. The counselor might also ask if the patient's partner or other family member is aware of the appointment and what their reactions were.

The American College of Medical Genetics (ACMG) maintains a list of genetic test results for medical conditions that they consider should be reported to patients who undergo genetic testing (Kalia et al. 2017). Note that ACMG does not suggest that these conditions should always be tested for; rather, they are medically actionable conditions that may be detected incidentally when a patient undergoes a panel test or, more likely, a exome/genome screen. Currently the list stands at fifty-nine conditions, but it is regularly updated and amended. Patients who are undergoing a test that may include any of these conditions should be told upfront that while certainly they have every right not to know this information, practice guidelines recommend that the results be disclosed. This would be an opportunity to explore with patients why they would or would not want to hear certain information.

A DIAGNOSIS IS NOT THE END OF THE ODYSSEY

The "diagnostic odyssey" is what we call that meandering, lengthy, and frustrating quest for a diagnosis. Genetic counselors, medical geneticists, and patients with rare disorders and their families are achingly familiar with it. The allusion to Homer's *Odyssey* is apt. Odysseus's decade of wandering was replete with perils, disappointment, love, wonder, whimsical gods, adventure, and frustration. Surely *some* specialist *somewhere* in the world can tell me what condition my child has been born with! Genetic testing technologies like exome/genome sequencing have shortened the quest for many patients, though perhaps not as often as we would hope.

The label "diagnostic odyssey" suggests that the diagnosis is the end of the odyssey, and therein lies the problem: Many families and patients discover that a diagnosis does not necessarily allow them to settle down and get on with their lives. A successful diagnostic workup may be the end of the odyssey for clinicians, but for patients and families the diagnostic quest is just one phase in the life cycle of genetic disorders.

A diagnosis may answer some questions such as cause and recurrence risk, but it can also create a whole new set of issues. For patients diagnosed with ultra-rare conditions, families may be faced with frustration from a lack of available knowledge about treatment or prognosis. Even if medical interventions are possible, finding and accessing those resources, and getting health insurers to pay for them, can be a major undertaking. Or a condition's rarity may make it impossible to form an effective patient/

family community to provide advocacy and support. The diagnostic odyssey may result in some patients feeling like diagnostic oddities.

If a newly diagnosed syndrome turns out to be untreatable or life-shortening, parents may lose all hope and descend into existential despair. A lack of diagnosis at least holds the glimmer of a chance that a treatment or cure is out there somewhere. Patients who have a diagnosis changed from a previous incorrect one may lose the sense of identity and support supplied by the disease community they had been involved with for years.

The label "diagnostic odyssey" focuses on one medical aspect of a condition. Clinicians can take much-deserved professional satisfaction in having finally solved a longstanding mystery. But for many families, living with a genetic condition is not a temporally demarcated event and, above all, is not only a medical experience. Patients will still need to implement strategies and solutions to the social, educational, lifestyle, and psychological ramifications of the disorder. It is an ongoing journey, one that continues to unfold as patients age and develop new symptoms, family structures evolve over time, medical treatment advances, and sociocultural changes reshape attitudes toward inclusivity and the availability of resources. A genetic condition, named or not, will continually present new challenges throughout a patient's entire life.

We do not mean to imply that a diagnosis is unimportant. We recognize the emotional and potential medical value of finally "putting a name on it." But the name just points families in new directions to unexplored regions with different threats, problems, and rewards. Genetic counselors need to continue to partner with patients and utilize their counseling skills and clinical knowledge to help guide patients and their families on their lifelong journeys.

REFERENCES

Athens, B. A., S. L. Caldwell, K. L. Umstead, P. D. Connors, E. Brenna, and B. B. Biesecker. 2017. "A Systematic Review of Randomized Controlled Trials to Assess Outcomes in Genetic Counseling." *Journal of Genetic Counseling* 26, no. 5: 902–33. doi:10.1007/s10897-017-0082-y.

Biesecker, B. B. 2018. "Genetic Counselors as Social and Behavioral Scientists in the Era of Precision Medicine." *American Journal of Medical Genetics C: Seminars in Medical Genetics* 178: 10–14. doi:10.1002/ajmg.c.31609.

Biesecker, B. B., K. L. Lewis, K. L. Umstead, J. J. Johnston, E. Turbitt, K. P. Fishler, . . . L. G. Biesecker. 2018. "Web Platform vs In-Person Genetic Counselor for Return of Carrier Results from Exome Sequencing: A Randomized Clinical Trial." *JAMA Internal Medicine* 178: 338–46. doi:10.1001/jamainternmed.2017.8049.

Brett, G. R., E. J. Wilkins, E. T. Creed, K. West, A. Jarmolowicz, G. M. Valente, . . . I. Macciocca. 2018. "Genetic Counseling in the Era of Genomics: What's All the Fuss about?" *Journal of Genetic Counseling* 27, no. 5: 1010–21. doi:10.1007/s10897-018-0216-x.

Cohen, S. A., M. L. Marvin, B. D. Riley, H. S. Vig, J. A. Rousseau, and S. L. Gustafson. 2013. "Identification of Genetic Counseling Service Delivery Models in Practice: A Report from the NSGC Service Delivery Model Task Force." *Journal of Genetic Counseling* 22, no. 4: 411–21. doi:10.1007/s10897-013-9588-0.

Colicchia, L. C., C. L. Holland, J. A. Tarr, D. M. Rubio, S. D. Rothenberger, and J. C. Chang. 2016. "Patient–Health Care Provider Conversations about Prenatal Genetic Screening: Recommendation or Personal Choice." *Obstetrics and Gynecology* 127, no. 6: 1145–52. doi:10.1097/AOG.0000000000001433.

Engels, A. C., P. DeKoninck, J. L. van der Merwe, T. Van Mieghem, P. Stevens, B. Power, . . . J. A. Deprest. 2013. "Does Website-Based Information Add Any Value in Counseling Mothers Expecting a Baby with Severe Congenital Diaphragmatic Hernia?" *Prenatal Diagnosis* 33, no. 11: 1027–32. doi:10.1002/pd.4190.

Gammon, B. L., S. A. Kraft, M. Michie, and M. Allyse. 2016. "'I Think We've Got Too Many Tests!': Prenatal Providers' Reflections on Ethical and Clinical Challenges in the Practice Integration of Cell-Free DNA Screening." *Ethics, Medicine and Public Health* 2, no. 3: 334–42. doi:10.1016/j.jemep.2016.07.006.

Gordon, E. S., D. Babu, and D. A. Laney. 2018. "The Future Is Now: Technology's Impact on the Practice of Genetic Counseling." *American Journal of Medical Genetics Part C* 178: 15–23 doi:10.1002/ajmg.c.31599.

Green, R. C., K. D. Christensen, L. A. Cupples, N. R. Relkin, P. H. Whitehouse, C. D. Royal, . . . J. S. Roberts, REVEAL Study Group. 2015. "A Randomized Noninferiority Trial of Condensed Protocols for Genetic Risk Disclosure of Alzheimer's Disease." *Alzheimer's & Dementia* 11: 1222–230.

Hayeems, R. Z., R. Babul-Hirji, N. Hoang, R. Weksberg, and C. Shuman. 2016. "Parents' Experience with Pediatric Microarray: Transferrable Lessons in the Era of Genomic Counseling." *Journal of Genetic Counseling* 25, no. 2: 298–304. doi:10.1007/s10897-015-9871-3.

Hooker, G. W., D. Babu, M. F. Myers, H. Zierhut, and M. McAllister. 2017. "Standards for the Reporting of Genetic Counseling Interventions in Research and Other Studies (GCIRS): An NSGC Task Force Report." *Journal of Genetic Counseling* 26: 355–60. doi:10.1007/s10897-017-0076-9.

Jones, G. E., J. H. Singletary, A. Cashmore, V. Jain, J. Abhulimhen, J. Chauhan, . . . J. G. Barwell. 2016. "Developing and Assessing the Utility of a YouTube-Based Clinical Genetics Video Channel for Families Affected by Inherited Tumours." *Familial Cancer* 15, no. 2: 351–55. doi:10.1007/s10689-016-9866-8.

Joseph, G., R. J. Pasick, D. Schillinger, J. Luce, C. Guerra, and J. K. Y. Cheng. 2017. "Information Mismatch: Cancer Risk Counseling with Diverse Underserved Patients." *Journal of Genetic Counseling* 26, no. 5: 1090–104. doi:10.1007/s10897-017-0089-4.

Kalia, S. S., K. Adelman, S. J. Bale, W. K. Chung, C. Eng, J. P. Evans, . . . D. T. Miller, on behalf of the ACMG Secondary Findings Maintenance Working Group. 2017. "Recommendations for Reporting of Secondary Findings in Clinical Exome and Genome Sequencing, 2016 Update (ACMG SF v2.0): A Policy Statement of the American College of Medical Genetics and Genomics." *Genetics in Medicine* 19: 249–55. doi:10.1038/gim.2016.190.

Kessler, S. 2001. "Psychological Aspects of Genetic Counseling XIV. Nondirectiveness and Counseling Skills." *Genetic Testing* 5: 187–91.

Knutzen, D. M., K. A. Stoll, D. W. McClellan, S. H. Deering, and L. M. Foglia. 2013. "Improving Knowledge about Prenatal Screening Options: Can Group Education Make a

Difference?" *Journal of Maternal, Fetal, and Neonatal Medicine* 26, no. 18: 1799–803. doi:10.3109/14767058.2013.804504.

Kurian, A. W., Y. Li, A. S. Hamilton, K. D. Ward, S. T. Hawley, M. Morrow, . . . S. J. Katz. 2017. "Gaps in Incorporating Germline Genetic Testing into Treatment Decision-Making for Early-Stage Breast Cancer." *Journal of Clinical Oncology* 35, no. 20: 2232–39. doi:10.1200/JCO.2016.71.6480.

Madlensky, L., A. M. Trepanier, D. Dragun, B. Lerner, K. M. Shannon, and H. Zierhut. 2017. "A Rapid Systematic Review of Outcome Studies in Genetic Counseling." *Journal of Genetic Counseling* 6, no. 3: 361–78. doi:10.1007/s10897-017-0067-x.

Mette, L. A., A. M. Saldívar, N. E. Poullard, I. C. Torres, S. G. Seth, B. H. Pollock, and G. E. Tomlinson. 2016. "Reaching High-Risk Underserved Individuals for Cancer Genetic Counseling by Video-Teleconferencing." *Journal of Community and Supportive Oncology* 14, no. 4:162–68. doi:10.12788/jcso.0247.

Patch, C., and A. Middleton. 2018. "Genetic Counselling in the Era of Genomic Medicine." *British Medical Bulletin* 126: 27–36. doi:10.1093/bmb/ldy008.

Peterson, E. B., W. S. Chou, A. Gaysynsky, M. Krakow, A. Elrick, M. J. Khoury, and K. A. Kaphingst. 2018. "Communication of Cancer-Related Genetic and Genomic Information: A Landscape Analysis of Reviews." *Translational Behavioral Medicine* 8, no. 1: 59–70. doi:10.1093/tbm/ibx063.

Ramos, E., and S. M. Weissman. 2018. "The Dawn of Consumer-Directed Testing." *American Journal of Medical Genetics Part C* 178: 89–97. doi:10.1002.ajmg.c.31603.

Stoll, K., S. Kubendran, and S. A. Cohen. 2018. "The Past, Present and Future of Service Delivery in Genetic Counseling: Keeping up in the Era of Precision Medicine." *American Journal of Medical Genetics* 178: 24–37. doi:10.1002/ajmg.c.31602.

Sweet, K., S. Hovick, A. C. Sturm, T. Schmidlen, E. Gordon, B. Bernhardt, L. Wawak, . . . M. Christman. 2016. "Counselees' Perspectives of Genomic Counseling Following Online Receipt of Multiple Actionable Complex Disease and Pharmacogenomic Results: A Qualitative Research Study." *Journal of Genetic Counseling* 26, no. 4: 738–51. doi:10.1007/s10897-016-0044-9.

Watson, C. H., M. Ulm, P. Blackburn, L. Smiley, M. Reed, R. Covington, . . . T. Tillmanns T. 2016. "Video-Assisted Genetic Counseling in Patients with Ovarian, Fallopian, and Peritoneal Carcinoma." *Gynecologic Oncology* 143: 109–12. doi:10.1016/j.ygyno.2016.07.094.

Weil, J., K. Ormond, J. Peters, K. Peters, B. B. Biesecker, and B. LeRoy. 2006. "The Relationship of Nondirectiveness to Genetic Counseling: Report of a Workshop at the 2003 NSGC Annual Education Conference." *Journal of Genetic Counseling* 15: 85–93.

Wolfe, C. R., V. F. Reyna, C. L. Widmer, E. M. Cedillos, C. R. Fisher, P. G. Brust-Renck, and A. M. Weil. 2015. "Efficacy of a Web-Based Intelligent Tutoring System for Communicating Genetic Risk of Breast Cancer: A Fuzzy-Trace Theory Approach." *Medical Decision Making* 35, no. 1: 46–59. doi:10.1177/0272989X14535983.

Woodson, A. H, J. L. Profato, M. Park, S. H. Rizvi, N. Elsayegh, A. G. Rieber, and B. K. Arun. 2015. "Service Delivery Model and Experiences in a Cancer Genetics Clinic for an Underserved Population." *Journal of Health Care for the Poor and Underserved* 26, no. 3: 784–91. doi:10.1353/hpu.2015.0090.

APPENDIX

Transcript of a Genetic Counseling Session

This hypothetical counseling session is intended to highlight some of the issues discussed in the text. As with most counseling sessions, the genetic counselor displays a mix of skills and weaknesses. It is not intended as a criticism of the genetic counselor; instead, it is meant to be a starting point for discussion about how the session was handled. Consider some of the things the counselor said, or didn't say, and think about how it might have been handled differently. What would you have said to or asked of the patient at various points in the session? What are some of the strengths of this counselor? What aspects of the counselor's skills need further work? What are good ways to try to reconcile a patient's religious beliefs with your scientific and clinical knowledge? How might your confidence and belief in the scientific worldview impair your ability to help devoutly religious patients to make good decisions and to understand the medical implications of their family history? Do you, deep down, feel that religious patients are ignoring scientific explanations at the peril of their own life and health? What are your own religious beliefs and do you have any problems reconciling those with your work as a genetic counselor?

The client, Tatiana, is a healthy thirty-eight-year-old woman who moved from Novosobirsk, Russia, to Portland, Oregon, twenty years ago with her parents and her two younger brothers. She and her husband are evangelical Christians. She is a married stay-at-home mother of a three-year-old daughter and lives near her nuclear family in Portland. Her expressive and receptive English skills are good. She has requested that no interpreter be used. She was referred by her gynecologist after she asked when she should start mammography because two paternal aunts, two female paternal first cousins, and her paternal grandmother have been diagnosed with breast cancer.

The counselor is a twenty-seven-year-old female born and raised in Boston who moved to Portland, Oregon, to accept a job as a cancer genetic counselor at a large private hospital. She graduated from her genetic counseling program two years ago. She is largely agnostic, but mostly hadn't given much thought to the role of religion in her life, in part because her family did not belong to a religious group. She is not currently in a committed relationship. She does not have children but figures that she will probably have a family at some point in the future.

The counselor has a typically busy day of meetings and patients and is running twenty-five minutes behind schedule at this point.

COUNS (A BIT HURRIEDLY AND DISTRACTED): Good morning, Tatiana. How are you today?

PT: I am good, but I am a bit worried about my daughter. I had to leave her with my brother's wife so I could come to this appointment. She is very attached to me and I am worried about how she will do without me. I like my sister-in-law, but she does not have children so I don't know if my daughter will be comfortable with her.

COUNS: Well, Tatiana, I am glad that you were able to make it today. We have some important things to discuss. But I will make sure that you get back to your daughter as soon as possible so she does not miss her mother too much.

PT: Thank you. My baby might get very upset if I am gone too long.

COUNS (*looking through the patient's chart and noticing out of the corner of her eye that a phone call is coming in on her desk phone; starts to think about the several patients she has been playing phone tag with*): So I understand that you are concerned about your family history?

PT: Well, I am here because my doctor told me I should make this appointment. I am not really sure why I am here and what you do. I have breast cancer in my family. But my relatives all smoked. And I don't think they really believed that God would help them.

COUNS: So you think that their smoking and lack of faith in God may have caused their breast cancer?

PT: God takes care of those who are true believers. My aunts said they believed in God, but I am not sure they really believed in him. If they really believed, they would not have smoked. Our bodies are God's temples and we are supposed to take care of ourselves.

COUNS: Tatiana, you bring up some very important issues. Tell me, what would you like to discuss today so I can make sure we make good use of your time?

PT: I pray to God every night that I don't get breast cancer and die like my aunt and my grandmother. I want to have more three children and I want to be around to take care of them.

COUNS: You are trying to be a good mother and I understand why your family history must worry you. Why don't you tell me a bit more about your family history?

PT: Well, what is important to know?

The counselor proceeds to take the patient's family history and learns that her paternal grandmother's sister died of "stomach cancer" in her early fifties, the cousins were both diagnosed with breast cancer in their thirties, and the other relatives were diagnosed in their sixties. The counselor realizes that it is not highly likely that they will be able to test an affected relative, based on what the patient told her about the complexity of the familial relationships and because one of the key relatives lives in Novosobirsk, Russia.

COUNS: Now that I know your family history better, I understand why your doctor sent you to me. She was concerned that there might be a genetic component to the breast cancer in your family and . . .

PT (*interrupts*): Please, what means "genetic component"?

COUNS: It means that there may an inherited predisposition to cancer in your family, and that might put you at higher risk of developing cancer, especially at a young age.

PT: Uh, what is "inheritable predisposition"?

COUNS (*pauses*): Well, family members sometimes look a bit alike. For example, you might have your mother's eye color, your father's nose, your grandmother's curly hair. In the same way that hair color or eye color runs in families, some diseases like cancer run in families too. Children are like a mix of their parents because they get some genetic material, what we call genes, from their mother and some from their father.

PT: This is good. I look nothing like my father, and his side of the family is where the cancer all is. I look just like my mother. I even laugh like she does. I have more of her what you call genes than my father's genes. This means I shouldn't get cancer. And I know that God will takes care of me. He wouldn't let me get cancer because I have a baby. And I don't smoke.

COUNS: Well, we are not always exactly like one parent or the other. Sometimes we may look or act more like one parent, but on the inside we can still be a bit different.

PT: This is true, I thinks I have my father's stomach. Neither of us can eat spicy food without getting an upset stomach. Oof.

COUNS (*smiles*): Yes, we get both the good and the bad from our parents, don't we? My family is the same way.

PT: Do you think God would give me cancer genes? Why would he do that?

COUNS: Maybe God sometimes works in complicated ways that can be hard for us to understand. In my job, I see a lot of suffering among some of my kindest, sweetest patients, and I can't always explain it.

PT: But all the answers are in the Bible, that is what I learned at church. I read it all the time. Don't you read the Bible?

COUNS: Sometimes, when it comes to genetics and medicine, the Bible may not tell us what we need to know.

PT: I think you are wrong. Maybe if you read your Bible more, you would know. You should come to my church sometimes. We welcome everyone.

COUNS: Thank you, I will think about that offer. You are right, there is probably more wisdom in the Bible than I realized. Tell me, do you think you might get breast cancer?

PT: Well, I guess, yes, it could happen. Maybe that is why I am came here today. To be honest, since I have had my baby, I worry a lot more. At my church they say that God sometimes gives us suffering so we can love him more. I think I should do something about this, but I don't want the doctor to cut off my breasts. I want to breastfeed my babies, and, besides, my husband would never let me do it. You seem very smart; tell me what I should do.

COUNS: You mention God a lot and you just told me about your church. Is religion very important to you?

PT: Yes, of course.

COUNS: Do you think that religion can help answer scientific questions?

PT: Religion, science, it is all God's works. God will answer all of our questions, if we pray at him.

COUNS: So you are a strong Christian? Tell me about your faith, Tatiana.

PT: All of us are sinners, and we can only be redeemed by our love of God and God's love for us. In Russia, where I was born, God is illegal. We are told that you can't believe in God. But my religion tries to spread God's word everywhere in Russia so everyone can know about him. The government does not want us to do this. That is why I am in the US now. My country told me I can't believe in God, so we moved here so we don't get thrown in the jail. I am not going to stop believing in God just because the government says so. You should be thankful that you can go to church every Sunday without worrying that the police will arrest you and then your family will never see you again.

COUNS: Yes, there is a lot more religious freedom in America than in many other countries. [*Pauses*]. Some Christian patients think that doctors are God's hands on earth when it comes to making medical decisions. Other patients think that they do not need to see a doctor, and that God will take care of all of their problems. What are your thoughts on this?

PT: Sometimes I am not so sure but I think that God put doctors here to help us, but if we stop praying and believing in God then even doctors can't help us. So maybe that is why I am here today.

COUNS: Well, I am glad that you came to see me. I think together we can come up with a plan that will help you stay as healthy as possible.

PT: Gods willing.

COUNS: I guess you have figured even before now that breast cancer may be running in your family and because of this you may be at higher risk of developing breast cancer. Has anyone ever mentioned breast cancer genetic testing to you?

PT: You mean likes that movie star, what is her name, Angelina Jolie? Didn't she cut off her breasts? So young! She was about my age. I am worried about cutting off the breasts.

COUNS: Well, there are a lot of different choices women can make about reducing their risk of developing breast cancer, but you don't have to make any of those choices yet. Let's talk first about how genetic testing might help you make some informed choices on down the road.

PT: Yes, you are right. Sometimes I worry so much about the cancer that I get—how you say—ahead of myself.

COUNS: Do you know much about genetic testing?

PT: No, I have never had any genetic tests and none of my friends have either. Tell me—is it difficult to get at my genes?

COUNS: Getting at your genes is the easy part. It is just a blood draw, or, if you prefer, we can take a sample of your saliva. The hard parts are figuring out if you should have testing, what is the best genetic test for you, and then interpreting the test results.

The counselor then proceeds to explain the background risks of breast cancer, the role of genetics and other factors in developing breast cancer, and the risks associated with BRCA mutations. She also discusses screening and risk-reducing strategies.

PT: So I have to have a genetic test today? Is that what you are telling me?

COUNS: Oh no, no, of course not. The purpose of meeting with me is to help you understand your risks and options better. Some women decide to have testing today, some decide to think about it for a while, and other women just choose to never have testing. It is all up to you. I am not going to make you do anything.

PT: You mean you won't give me any advice even?

COUNS: Well, I can help you figure out what is the best choice for you, but, Tatiana, I can't just tell you what to do.

PT: Will you tell me if I make a bad decision? This is very complicated, and I am not sure I can understand it enough to make a decision. And my English is not so good.

COUNS: A lot of women tell me the same things you are saying, but I think many of those women make very good choices, and I think you can too. By the way, you speak English very well.

PT: Okay then.

COUNS: Looking at your family history, a test you should think about is the BRCA test. This test looks for mutations in the BRCA1 and BRCA2 genes. If the test is positive, then it means that you have a much higher chance than average of getting breast and some other cancers.

PT: Okay, let's do the BRCA test then, if you think it is a goods test. But what is this mutation you are talking about? Like the X-Men?

COUNS: Well, it is a good test, but let me explain a bit more. But first let me ask you, your cousin and your aunt who have had breast cancer—have they had any genetic testing related to their breast cancer?

PT: No, my cousin in Russia, there is no genetic testing there. It is very hard to get to see a doctor even if you are sick. And my aunt, she lives in Washington state. But she and my father, they don't talk to each other. They have—what you call—family feud. They have not spoken for years. This is too bad, I thinks. But my aunt will not have anything to do with me.

COUNS: Well, we prefer to first test somebody in the family who has had cancer. It makes the test more accurate. Are you sure that you or somebody else in the family could not approach her about this? Sometimes I find that even for families who don't communicate, sometimes they are willing to temporarily call a truce and discuss health issues that might affect the whole family.

PT: No, I don't think that will happen.

COUNS: Okay, I understand. But I have to tell you that it can make it hard sometimes to interpret your results, especially if your testing is normal.

PT: I don't think I understand that. If my genetic test is normal, then I don't have the gene, right? Then I don't have to worry so much about cancer.

COUNS: Well, I wish I could say that. But there are many families like yours where all the genetic testing is normal.

PT: So that means their cancer was caused by cigarette smoking or air pollution or stress maybe. In Russia, we have lots of air pollution and everybody smokes. Maybe that is what caused all the cancer sickness in my family.

COUNS: Hmmm, you are right. The environment can cause some kinds of cancer sometimes. But scientists and doctors also think that we haven't yet discovered all the genes linked to breast cancer. If your genetic test is negative, it could also mean that you have a gene that we just haven't discovered yet. But if we found a BRCA gene mutation in your aunt, and you didn't inherit it, then we could say that, for your family, BRCA is the cause of the breast cancer and because you don't have it, then you are not at higher risk of breast cancer.

PT: You mean that if my aunt had a positive mutation, and mine was normal, I could not get cancer? God would be smiling on me then.

COUNS: Well, we have to be careful here. It wouldn't mean that you couldn't get cancer. It just means that you would face the average cancer risks that any woman faces.

PT: Ugh. I wish my aunt would have testing. But I know I cannot talk to her at all. She would not listen to me, and my father would be mad that I even tried to talks to her.

COUNS: Is there anybody else in the family who you could talk to and who might then talk to your aunt? Does she have any daughters, a cousin of yours, maybe you could approach?

PT: No, her daughter died from the breast cancer. My aunt has been very different since then, not the same person. Are you sure you can't just test me?

COUNS: Yes, we can do that. If the test is positive, then we know what it means. But if your test is negative, we think you may still be at higher breast cancer risk because you could have a "mystery" gene.

PT: Oh right, you said that before. Still, I will take a chance. If I am a mutant, well, at least I would have a better idea of my risk and what to do about it. But if I have the gene, I am definitely going to get cancer, right?

COUNS: No, no. Genes don't work like that. If your test is positive, then you are at a higher risk of getting cancer, and the doctors will suggest some ways to lower your risks or, if you get cancer, to find it when it is still very small and hasn't spread. Once cancer has spread, it is a lot harder to treat.

PT: Couldn't I just eat better and exercise more? Everybody eats at fast food and sits around their living rooms like they are, how you say it, couch potatoes? No wonder there is so much cancer.

COUNS: So far, most studies say that when breast cancer has a strong genetic component, your diet and lifestyle may not lower your risk enough.

PT: You mean I don't have to worry about what I eat? I will get cancer anyway?

COUNS: No, I am sorry, I wasn't clear. A healthy diet and exercise are important, especially for reducing your chances of serious illnesses like diabetes and heart disease. And if you are healthy to begin with, it is easier for your body to recover from cancer and chemotherapy.

PT: So this BRCA test, I think I want it. But I don't know if God wants me to have it.

COUNS: How would you know if God wants you to have the test or not?

PT: I am not sure. Maybe I would just know it. If God wants me to have it, then he would let me know it.

COUNS: We should talk about the cost of genetic testing and insurance coverage. It can be an expensive test. That can help some people decide if they want the test.

PT: Sometimes God . . . My family is not rich. We cannot pay for this test. You mean my insurance will not cover it? My doctor wants me to have it. So my insurance has to cover it, right?

COUNS: With your family history, there is a good chance that your insurance will cover genetic testing. But I can't say that for sure, and I don't know if they would cover all of the cost or just part of it.

PT: Well, if insurance doesn't cover it, maybe that is a sign from God that I shouldn't have the test.

COUNS: Maybe. But fortunately, the labs that I work with will check the coverage for you. If your insurance doesn't cover the test, then they will not run it without your permission.

PT: Can we trust the lab to do that? What if they make a mistake? My husband and I do not make much money, and we could not pay for it ourselves.

COUNS: I understand. But I have been working with these labs for a few years, and so far none of my patients have had a problem. And many of them have the same insurance as you.

PT: Well, I don't know. I am still worried. If my insurance doesn't cover it but the lab runs the test anyway, I will not pay their bill when they send it to me.

COUNS: I can't encourage you to not pay your bills. But I tell you what, if you get a large bill from the lab, and they had not warned you about that before they ran the test, let me know and I will straighten it out with them.

PT: Yes, I would like that.

COUNS: If you have the test, it usually takes about three weeks for the results to come back. Sometimes a little longer, sometimes a little shorter, it's hard to say for sure. But most of my patients hear back in no more than three weeks. How would you like me to notify you of the results?

PT: Notify me? I haven't even decided if I want to have the test yet!

COUNS: I'm sorry, Tatiana, you're right. I am jumping the gun, aren't I?

PT: I still don't know if the test is the right thing to do for me. I need to pray about it.

COUNS: Would it help if you spoke with your husband about this? Or a good friend?

PT: Well, that might help. But if God wants me to have or not have the test then he will tell me. That is more important than what my husband thinks.

COUNS: Do you think you need more information about the test? There are some things we haven't really discussed yet that might help you decide.

PT: You could tell me some more. But I don't know if it would help me decide if it doesn't help me know God's wishes. What do you think I should do?

COUNS: Well, I can't make that decision for you. That is something you have to decide in your own way.

PT: But you're an expert. You should tell me what to do.

COUNS: It's true that I am an expert, but I am a medical expert. You are the best expert about yourself. And for you, this is a choice between you and God, not between you and me.

PT: True, but I don't want to do the *wrong* thing.

COUNS: I understand your worry. But I don't think there is a wrong choice for you. Having or not having the test are both a balance of good and bad and you should weigh the good and the bad for each choice. But don't worry, I will let you know if I think you make a *bad* decision, and why I think it might be a bad decision for you. Sometimes people make bad decisions because they don't want to admit that they don't fully understand all this technical information. If I think the decision you make is based on you not fully understanding the information, I will try to clarify that for you. But it is as much a decision of your heart as of your mind.

PT: I feel so much pressure to make this decision.

COUNS: This is an important decision for you, but it is not an urgent decision. You don't have cancer right now, and so it is not a matter of life and death. You don't have to rush into it. You can make the decision today, next week, next month, or even next year. Maybe the only bad decision here is a decision you rush into without considering everything carefully. Give yourself some breathing room if you need it.

PT: But I don't want to get cancer.

COUNS: Well, even if you were to have a positive genetic test, there is a pretty good chance you don't have cancer right now, and the odds are you wouldn't get cancer in the next few years. As a starting point, maybe you should consider having a mammogram soon. If the mammogram is normal, which it probably will be, then you might feel a little bit less pressure and worry.

PT: Yes, maybe that is good thing to do. But I have never had a mammogram. Do they hurt?

COUNS: Most women find them uncomfortable and not very pleasant but they don't take very long and usually women find the experience bearable.

PT: I hope it is not as painful as having a baby. Oof! That hurt a lot.

COUNS: I have never had a baby but I am pretty sure a mammogram is a lot less painful—and a lot quicker—than giving birth.

PT: That is good. I will ask my doctor about getting the mammogram.

The patient is now quiet for a few moments, and not looking directly at the counselor, apparently gathering her thoughts. After pausing for a bit, the counselor resumes.

COUNS: What are you thinking about right now? Have I confused you with too much information?

PT: Well, I was praying a bit because I am a bit confused but not because I don't understand what you said to me. I see why this testing might be helpful. But for some reason, I can't seem to say to myself that I want it. I was hoping God would give me an answer.

COUNS: I usually don't tell my patients what they should be doing. But, honestly, you sound to me like somebody who is not quite ready to make the decision to have a test today. I think you should not have a test today but keep open the possibility of having the test. Maybe in a few days, a few weeks, or even a few months or more you may feel ready to make the decision.

PT: Yes, I think you are right. I think my husband and I should pray together about this. And I will ask my church to pray for me. Praying opens up my heart to God, and then he will tell me the right thing to do. And maybe I will ask my doctor about that mammogram too.

COUNS: You know, Tatiana, I think that is a very good way to proceed. Do you need to talk some more about this now?

PT: No, thanks. You have told me everything I need to know. You have been very helpful. I hope you are not mad that I didn't have the test.

COUNS: Goodness, no, I am not mad. I am happy that I could help you figure out how you want to make your decision.

PT: Can I call you if I have questions or if I want to have the genetic test?

COUNS: Yes, of course, call me as often as you need to.

PT: Thanks you so much. Now I have to go home to my baby!

INDEX

Boxes are indicated by *b* following the page number.

For the benefit of digital users, indexed terms that span two pages (e.g., 52–53) may, on occasion, appear on only one of those pages.

ABGC. *See* American Board of Genetic Counseling
ABMG (American Board of Medical Genetics), 14
abortion, 12–13, 62–63, 96, 160, 188
accreditation, 14–15, 28
Accreditation Council for Genetic Counseling (ACGC), 16, 174
ACMG (American College of Medical Genetics), 112–13, 197
ACMS (American College of Medical Specialties), 14
adaptation, 33–34
   assistance during process of, 30–32
   cognitive adaptation theory, 34–35
   psychological wherewithal to adapt, 2, 34
adolescents, 56–57, 59
advocacy and advocacy groups, 25–26, 33–34, 89, 139, 181, 197–98
African American patients and clients
   sickle cell trait and insurance, 98
   trust of medical system, 47–48
age, 56–59
   adolescents, 56–57, 59
   age difference between counselor and patient/client, 58
   counselors' personal and familial experiences, 58–59
   older patients and accompanying family members, 57
   older patients and assessment of genetic risks for family, 57
   older patients and multiple health issues, 57
   young adults with parents present, 61–62
Allan, William, 9, 10–11
All of Us research program, 183
Alzheimer disease, 190–91
American Board of Genetic Counseling (ABGC)
   conflicts of interest, 111
   establishment of, 14–15
   practice-based competencies, 27–28, 29
   training requirements, 16
American Board of Medical Genetics (ABMG), 14
American College of Medical Genetics (ACMG), 112–13, 197
American College of Medical Specialties (ACMS), 14
American College of Obstetricians and Gynecologists, 191–92
American Eugenics Society, 10–11
American Journal of Human Genetics, 10–11
American Journal of Medical Genetics, 11
American Psychological Association, 144–45

(*211*)

American Society of Human Genetics
    (ASHG), 16–17
  definition of genetic counseling,
    19, 26–27
  official journal of, 10–11
Amish patients and clients, 50–51
amniocentesis, 12–14, 51–52
aneuploidy screening, 13–14, 191–92
Annals of Eugenics, 10
Annals of Human Genetics, 10
ASHG. *See* American Society of Human
    Genetics
"Asilomar meetings," 16
assertiveness training, 97–98
Association of Genetics Nurses and
    Counsellors, 121
Athens, Barbara A., 178
atomic bomb, 7
audio-recording of sessions,
    43–44, 82, 83
Austin, Jehannine, 21, 144–45
Australasian Society of Genetic
    Counsellors, 121

Backdoor to Eugenics (Duster), 24–25
Bebeau, M. J., 103
behavior modification, 152–53
Belmont Report, The, 97
Benoit, L. G., 79
bereavement counseling, 167, 168*b*
Biesecker, Barbara B., 28, 29, 173
bioethics. *See* ethics and bioethics
bipolar disorder, 55–56
Black, Rita Beck, 11–12
Boston Globe, 114
Bowman Gray School of Medicine, 9
BRCA testing
  counselors' personal and familial
    experiences, 58–59
  countertransference issues, 58
  cross-cultural issues, 47–48
  ethical approaches, 92, 93–94,
    98, 99–100
  feminist ethics, 96
  feminist therapy, 158
  immediacy, 139–40

  men and, 53
  problem-solving interventions,
    172, 181–82
  research led by genetic
    counselors, 172
  transcript of sample
    session, 201–9
breast cancer. *See also* BRCA testing
  age and, 56, 59
  conflicts of interest, 115, 119
  feminist therapy, 158
  nontraditional gender
    identification, 54
  paternal lineage, 53
  patients *vs.* clients, 44–45
  race and, 47–48
  transcript of sample session, 201–9

Canadian Association of Genetic
    Counselors, 121
case analysis process, 102–3, 103*b*
casuistry, 97
  counselor's application of, 97
  theoretical scenario and, 97
Catholic patients and clients, 62–63
CBT. *See* cognitive-behavioral therapy
    theories
Centers for Disease Control
    and Prevention
    (CDC), 21, 22*b*
Chaucer, Geoffrey, 43–44
chemotherapy, 55, 102, 105*b*
chorionic villus sampling, 13–14
chronic pain, 56
Civil Rights Act of 1964, 51–52
Clarke, A., 89
client-centered care, 27–28
  commitment to, 71
  counselors' personal and familial
    experience, 84
  crisis counseling *vs.,* 166
  goals of genetic counseling, 30–35
  patient/clients' values, 72
clients. *See* patients and clients;
    relational genetic counseling
Clinical Genetics, 11

Clinical Sequencing Exploratory
    Research (CSER), 171–72
closed-ended questions, 131
codes of ethics, 120–22
   binding nature of, 121
   definition of, 120–21
   NSGC, 121–22
   other organizations, 121
cognitive-behavioral therapy (CBT)
      theories, 150–53, 168b
   application to genetic
      counseling, 151–53
   theoretical concepts, 151
   theory strengths, 151
COIs. *See* conflicts of interest
Comfort, Nathaniel, 8, 9
compassion fatigue, 79–80
concreteness, 77, 138, 140
conflicts of interest (COIs), 111–20
   critical nature of, 114–15
   definition of, 111
   forms of, 112–13
      institutional COI, 113
      intangible financial COI, 113
      personal COI, 113
      professional COI, 113
      tangible financial COI, 112–13
   key concepts, 115–18
      conscious process, 115–16
      ethical fading, 117–18
      guidelines and training, 117
      motivated blindness, 118
      norm for human
         behavior, 116–17
      part of professional growth and
         development, 117
      unconscious/subconscious
         process, 116, 118
   NSGC resources, 112
   perceived, 118–20
      examples of, 119–20
   real *vs.* potential, 113–14
Contergan (Grippex;
      thalidomide), 9–10
contracting, 127–28, 129
Coon, Carleton, 10–11

Cornelia de Lange
      syndrome, 31–32
Counseling Video Project, 173
countertransference. *See* transference
      and countertransference
Cowley, Lorraine, 100
crisis counseling, 165–66, 168b
   challenges of, 166
   identifying crises, 165
   patients/clients in crisis, 166
   strategies for, 165–66
CSER (Clinical Sequencing Exploratory
      Research), 171–72
culture. *See* race, ethnicity,
      and culture

Darwin, Charles, 8
deontology, 93–94
   confidentiality and, 94
   counselor's application of, 93
   motivations *vs.* consequences, 93–94
   premises of, 93
   theoretical scenario and, 93–94
de Shazer, Steve, 153
"diagnostic odyssey," 91, 197–98
Dice, Lee, 9, 10–11
Dickens, Charles, 1
Dight, Charles, 9
Dight Institute of Human Genetics, 9
Djurdjinovic, Luba, 18
Dor Yeshorim program, 63
Draper, Wickliffe, 10–11
Duchenne muscular dystrophy
      (DMD), 168b
Duster, Troy, 24–25
dysmorphology, 9–10, 50–51

East Asian patients and clients, 51
Ellis, Albert, 150
embryopathy, 9–10
Emery, Alan, 11–12
empathic understanding, 31–32,
      136–37, 138–39, 140, 149
enmeshment, 161, 163
Epstein, Charles, 17, 24–25
Erby, L. A., 173

ethics and bioethics, 3, 89–107
    approaching with humility, 90–91
    case deliberation, 100–3
        analysis of consequences, 107b
        case analysis process, 102–3, 103b, 106–7
        clarification of facts, 101–2
        consideration of all interested parties, 105b
        points of conflict, 104b
        qualification as dilemma, 100–1
    changing consensus, 91
    codes of ethics, 120–22
        binding nature of, 121
        definition of, 120–21
        NSGC, 121–22
        other organizations, 121
    conflicts of interest, 111–20
        critical nature of, 114–15
        definition of, 111
        forms of, 112–13
        key concepts, 115–18
        NSGC resources, 112
        perception of, 118–20
        real *vs.* perceived *vs.* potential, 113–14
    decision-making frameworks, 91–100
        casuistry, 97
        deontology, 93–94
        feminist ethics, 96–97
        principilism, 97–100
        strengths and weaknesses of, 92
        theoretical scenario, 92–93
        utilitarian theories, 94–95
        virtue ethics, 95–96
    definition of bioethics, 90
    evaluation criteria, 103–7
        analysis of consequences, 106
        consideration of all interested parties, 105–6
        obligations of all involved, 106, 107b
        points of conflict, 104
    examples of ethical dilemmas and divides, 89
ethnicity. *See* race, ethnicity, and culture
eugenics, 8–9
    changing ethical values, 91
    connection to genetic counseling, 15
    criticisms, 9, 15, 24–25, 89
    direct influence on medical genetics, 9
    geneticists' support for goals of, 9
    journals, 10–11
    origin of, 8
    separation of medical genetics from, 9
    Treasury of Human Inheritance, The (Pearson), 8–9
Eugenics Quarterly, 10
Eunpu, Deborah, 12, 18
experiential learning theory, 76–77

family dynamics, 59–62
    complex pedigrees, 59–60
    counselor's preconceived notions, 61
    dual function of pedigrees, 60
    fluid relationships, 60
    focus on women, 60–61
    older patients and family members, 57
    young adults with parents present, 61–62
family therapy, 161–63, 168b
    application to genetic counseling, 162–63
    theoretical concepts, 161
    theory-based interventions, 162
    theory strengths, 162
feminist ethics, 96–97
    disability advocacy and, 96
    premise of, 96
    prenatal diagnosis and, 96
    theoretical scenario and, 96–97
feminist theories, 155–58, 168b
    application to genetic counseling, 157–58
    theoretical concepts, 156
    theory-based interventions, 156–57
    theory strengths, 156
Folkman, S., 180–82

Fragile X syndrome, 99
Francis Galton Laboratory for National Eugenics, 8

Galton, Francis, 8
GCOS (Genetic Counseling Outcome Scale), 37, 173
Gelsinger, Jesse, 113
gender, 52–55
  feminist ethics, 96–97
    disability advocacy and, 96
    premise of, 96
    prenatal diagnosis and, 96
    theoretical scenario and, 96–97
  feminist theories, 155–58
    application to genetic counseling, 157–58
    theoretical concepts, 156
    theory-based interventions, 156–57
    theory strengths, 156
  focus on women, 53, 60–61
  interpreters, 51–52
  LGBQT+ patients and clients, 54–55
  men's participation in genetic counseling, 52–53
  Muslim patients and clients, 51
  transference and counter transference, 54
genetic counseling. See also genetic counseling research; genetic counselors; history of genetic counseling; patients and clients; relational genetic counseling
  active partnership vs. reassuring platitudes, 32–33
  assumptions underlying, 2
  avoiding normalization or minimization, 33–34
  client-centered care, 30–35
  defining, 2–3, 19, 193
    ASHG, 26–27
    CDC's description, 21, 22b
    definitional evolution, 24–30
    in era of genomic medicine, 192–94

NSGC's practice definition, 29–30
proposed practice definition (Resta and Biesecker), 28–29
educational model, 22–23, 145–46
genetic diagnosis and medical management vs., 27
genetic testing vs., 1–2
goals of, 1–2, 30–36, 125
  adult, 35
  common diseases, 35–36
  pediatric, 35
  prenatal, 35
nondirectiveness, 24, 140–41, 147–48
origin of term, 10–11
patient/client outcomes, 36–37
practice-based competencies, 27–28, 29
prevention issues, 24–26
psychoeducational model, 21, 23, 28–29, 34–35
psychotherapeutic model, 11–12, 21, 22, 144–45
Reciprocal Engagement Model (REM), 126
transcript of sample session, 201–9
Genetic Counseling (Journal de Génétique Humaine), 18
Genetic Counseling (Kessler), 24–25
Genetic Counseling Outcome Scale (GCOS), 37, 173
genetic counseling research, 4, 171–83
  contribution genetic counselors make to, 171–72, 172b
  doctoral training, 176–77
  key gaps in, 178–79
  led by genetic counselors, 172–73
  need for evidence-based practice, 174–76
  as a priority for the profession, 172b, 173–74
  qualitative methods, 175–76
  quantitative methods, 175
  research training, 172b
  systematic literature reviews, 174–75
  theoretically informed research, 179–82
  translational genomics and, 182–83

genetic counselors. *See also* relational genetic counseling
  advocating course of action, 76
  approaching ethical dilemmas with humility, 90–91
  assumptions about patient/clients' needs, 74–75
  audio-recording of sessions, 43–44, 82, 83
  compassion fatigue, 79–80
  considering what patients/clients already know, 75, 76–78
  counseling conducted by medical geneticists *vs.*, 11
  counseling experiences, 84–85
  developing unique but adaptable style, 5
  educating patients/clients, 74
  heightening sensitivity to client characteristics, 43
  issue of name, 17
  lack of diversity among, 48, 62, 69
  learning styles, 77–78
  lecture approach, 72–73
  needs of client and context as guidance in education, 75–76
  obligations of, 107b
  outcome studies, 36
  overly technical, scientific, abstract language, 72–73, 77, 131–32
  personal experiences, 58–59, 80–81, 83–84
  preconceived notions, biases, and stereotypes, 45–47, 48, 50, 61, 78–79
  presenting new information, 76–77
  professional burnout, 79–80
  professional supervision, 43–44, 81, 82–85, 141
  psychological profile and makeup of, 3, 69–85
    control, 70
    emotional intelligence, 69
    enthusiasm for science, 72–73, 74–75
    moral and political beliefs of, 71
    optimism, 69
    patient education, 74–78
    personal beliefs of, 72–73
    respect and value for patients/clients, 70, 71, 74
    self-awareness and self-knowledge, 2, 3, 43–44, 80–83
    tolerance for uncertainty, 70
    value-neutral care *vs.* value-laden decisions, 72
  skills of, 1
  support services, 81
  tailoring education to patient/clients' literacy, 74
  typological thinking, 45–46
Genetics and Medicine Historical Network, 8
genograms, 162–63
genomic medicine, genetic counseling in era of, 4, 187–98
  diagnosis and "diagnostic odyssey," 197–98
  enhancing psychological outcomes, 192
  multigene panels and sequencing, 188–89, 195
  multiplex genetic testing, 193
  outcomes of pre-test genetic counseling, 190–91
  potential decline of pre-test genetic counseling, 190, 191, 194
  role of genetic counselors, 189
  service delivery models, 194–95
  which results to share with patients/clients, 195–97
Gorlin, Robert, 8
Grippex (thalidomide; Contergan), 9–10
group therapy, 158–61
  application to genetic counseling, 160–61
  theoretical concepts, 158–59
  theory-based interventions, 159–60
  theory strengths, 159

Harper, Peter, 8
Health Belief Model (HBM), 179–80

health/medical status, 55–56
Heimler, Audrey, 18
Heredity Clinic, 9
Herndon, C. Nash, 9, 10–11
Hesse-Biber, S., 96
Hispanic and Latino patients and clients, 51–52
history of genetic counseling, 2, 7–19, 188
 accreditation, 14–15
 "Asilomar meetings," 16
 conducted by medical geneticists *vs.* genetic counselors, 11
 eugenics and, 8–9, 15
 expansion of opportunities, 13–14
 integration of counseling skills, 12
 integration of psychological component, 11–12
 journals, 10–11
 medical genetics and, 7–8, 9–10, 12–15, 17
 professional society, 14–15, 16–19
 social trends, 12–13
 training programs, 13, 15–16
Holmes, Samuel J., 10–11
Hooton, Ernest, 10–11
Huntington disease, 55–56, 89

India's Board of Genetic Counseling, 121
informed consent, 51, 57, 95–96
Injeyan, M. C., 79
insurance coverage, 188–89, 193, 197–98
 African American patients and clients, 98
 gender and, 53, 54–55
 LGBQT+ patients and clients, 54–55
interpreters, 51–52
Introduction to Medical Genetics (Robert), 9

Johns Hopkins University, 10, 82
Journal of Genetic Counseling, 10, 18, 30, 172, 174
Journal of Medical Genetics, 11

Kessler, Seymour, 11–12, 21, 22, 24–25, 82, 140–41
Kevles, Daniel, 8
Klass, Phyllis, 18
Kolb, David, 76–77

language, 51–52
Lazarus, R. S., 180–82
LGBQT+ patients and clients
 body image, 54–55
 complexity of risks and treatments, 54
 coverage of treatment, 54–55
Lilienthal, Evelyn, 18
Lindee, Susan, 7
Lippman, Abby, 23
logorrhea, 55–56
Lucassen, A., 94
Lynch syndrome, 100, 102, 104*b*, 105*b*, 107*b*

Macklin, Madge, 10–11
Mand, C., 93
Marks, Joan, 13
McAllister, Marion, 37, 173
McConkie-Rosell, A., 93
McKusick, Victor, 10
medical genetics, 7–8, 9–10
 counseling conducted by medical geneticists *vs.* genetic counselors, 11
 first clinic, 9
 groundbreaking textbooks, 9
 influence of eugenics on, 9
 journals, 10–11
 Mendelian Inheritance in Man (McKusick), 9–10
 rubella and thalidomide birth defect epidemics, 9–10
 separation from eugenics, 9
 separation of genetic counseling as independent profession, 13–15, 17
Mendelian Inheritance in Man (McKusick), 10
Mental Retardation and Congenital Malformations of the Central Nervous System (Warkany), 8

methylphenidate (Ritalin), 55–56
MTHFR gene testing, 112–13
Muslim patients and clients, 51

National Fragile X Foundation, 99
National Geographic, 48
National Human Genome Research Institute, 82
National Institutes of Health, 171–72
National Society of Genetic Counselors (NSGC)
   client and patient outcomes, 22, 36–37
   Code of Ethics, 112, 121–22
   conflicts of interest, 112
   contracting, 127–28
   Ethics Advisory Group, 122
   Ethics Subcommittee, 102–3, 121
   feminist ethics, 96
   formation of, 18
   issue of name, 17
   Journal of Genetic Counseling, 18
   membership criteria, 18
   mission of, 18
   national representation, 18
   practice definition, 29
   reporting standards, 191
   research, 173
   values and beliefs of counselors, 71
   workforce study, 178
Native American patients and clients, 49–50
Nazi Germany and World War II, 9, 91
neural tube defects
   folic acid, 25
   maternal serum screening, 13–14
New York Times, 114
nondirectiveness, 24, 140–41, 147–48
NSGC. *See* National Society of Genetic Counselors

Office for Civil Rights Policy Guidance, 51–52
OMIM (*Online Mendelian Inheritance in Man*), 10

online genetic counseling and tele-genetic counseling, 174–75, 178–79, 194–95
ornithine transcarbamylase deficiency, 113
Osborn, Frederick, 10–11
ovarian cancer, 119–20, 190–91
   feminist therapy, 158
   nontraditional gender identification, 54
   paternal lineage, 53

paraphrasing, 82–83, 133–35, 136, 137
Parker, M., 94
Patient-Reported Outcome (PRO) research, 173
patients and clients. *See also* relational genetic counseling
   affective and cognitive responses to genetic information, 23–24, 30–32, 53, 75–76, 145–46
   avoiding lecture approach with, 72–73
   characteristics of, 3, 43–63
      age, 56–59
      family dynamics, 59–62
      gender, 52–55
      health/medical status, 55–56
      language, 51–52
      race, ethnicity, and culture, 47–51
      religion and spirituality, 62–63
   desire to "know everything they can," 75
   difference between patients and clients, 44–45
   educating, 74–78
   goodness of, 2, 72
   handling multiple causal attributions, 32
   learning styles, 76–77
   parents holding themselves responsible for child's condition, 32
   psychological impact and adaptation, 2, 22, 30–32, 33–35, 145–46

tailoring education to science/health
literacy of, 74
terminology for, 44–45
uniqueness of, 2, 3
which results to share with, 195–97
Patterson, C. H., 125, 136–37, 138
Paul, Diane, 8, 9
Pearson, Karl, 8–9, 10
person-centered theory, 146–50, 168*b*
application to genetic
counseling, 149–50
theoretical concepts, 148
theory-based interventions, 149
theory strengths, 148–49
Pindborg, Jens, 8
planned behavior theory, 180
Potter, Van Rensselaer, 90
prenatal genetic counseling, 9, 13–14,
191–92, 195
affective and cognitive responses to
genetic information, 23
client safety and trust, 126–27, 128
cognitive-behavioral therapy, 151–52
criticism of, 89, 91, 96, 191
establishing relationships, 130
feminist theories, 157–58
focus on women, 60–61
goal of, 35
nondirectiveness, 147–48
religion and spirituality, 62–63
prevention issues
avoiding birth of affected
fetuses, 24–25
birth defect prevention goal,
24–25, 26
disparities in access to services, 25–26
inclusion of those with
disabilities, 25–26
informed choice and differing
views, 24–26
principilism, 97–100
autonomy, 97–98
beneficence, 99
counselor's application of, 100
justice, 99–100
nonmaleficence, 98–99

theoretical scenario and, 98, 99–100
Principles of Bioethics, The (Beauchamp
and Childress), 97
Principles of Heredity (Snyder), 9
PRO (Patient-Reported Outcome)
research, 173
problem-solving (solution-focused)
therapy, 153–55, 168*b*
application to genetic counseling, 155
theoretical concepts, 153
theory-based interventions, 154–55
theory strengths, 153–54
professional burnout, 79–80
prostate cancer, 54
psychoeducational model, 21, 23
affective and cognitive responses to
genetic information, 23–24
practice definition, 28–29
"Psychological Aspects of Genetic
Counseling" (Kessler), 12
*Psychological Aspects of Genetic
Counselling* (Emery), 11–12
psychological aspects of genetic
diagnoses, 2, 27–28, 52, 98–99,
189–90, 192, 194
early exploration of and training in,
11–12, 15–16
family dynamics, 60–61
psychological counseling theories,
4, 143–68
bereavement counseling, 167
cognitive-behavioral therapy, 150–53
application to genetic
counseling, 151–53
theoretical concepts, 151
theory strengths, 151
crisis counseling, 165–66
family therapy, 161–63
application to genetic
counseling, 162–63
theoretical concepts, 161
theory-based interventions, 162
theory strengths, 162
feminist theories, 155–58
application to genetic
counseling, 157–58

psychological counseling theories (*cont.*)
   theoretical concepts, 156
   theory-based interventions, 156–57
   theory strengths, 156
  group therapy, 158–61
   application to genetic
    counseling, 160–61
   theoretical concepts, 158–59
   theory-based
    interventions, 159–60
   theory strengths, 159
  guiding counseling by means
   of, 144–47
  person-centered theory, 147–50
   application to genetic
    counseling, 149–50
   theoretical concepts, 148
   theory-based interventions, 149
   theory strengths, 148–49
  problem-solving (solution-focused)
   therapy, 153–55
   application to genetic
    counseling, 155
   theoretical concepts, 153
   theory-based interventions, 154–55
   theory strengths, 153–54
  quality of therapeutic alliance, 146
  strength-based counseling, 164
   application to genetic
    counseling, 164
   theoretical concepts, 164
  time limitations, 146
Psychological Genetic Counseling
  (Weil), 12
psychotherapeutic model, 11–12, 21, 22, 144–45
psychotherapy
  APA definition of, 144–45
  client and patient outcomes, 36
  for genetic counselors, 141
  integration of into genetic
   counseling, 11–12

race, ethnicity, and culture, 47–48
  approaching ethical dilemmas with
   humility, 91

awkward situations, 49–50
compassion fatigue, 80
cultural knowledge, 48–51
language, 51–52
of most genetic counselors, 48
nonadherence with medication
  usage, 48
past experiences with health care
  and, 47–48
socioeconomic status and, 47–48
study of ethnocultural issues, 15–16
Race Implicit Association Test, 50
reasoned action theory, 180
Reciprocal Engagement Model (REM), 36–37, 126
Recognizable Patterns of Human
  Malformation (Smith), 8
Reed, Sheldon, 9, 10–11
relational genetic counseling, 3–4, 125–41
  client safety and trust, 126–29
   contracting, 127–28
   realistic effort to provide, 126–27
   time limitations, 127
  closed-ended questions, 131
  concreteness, 138
  empathic understanding, 136–37
  establishing relationships, 129–31
  genuineness, 138
  paraphrasing, 133–35
  providing information, 131–33, 132*b*
   ensuring relevant information is
    understood, 133
   standardized protocols for, 132*b*, 132–33
  reflection of feelings, 135–36
  respect, 138
  therapeutic Interventions, 138–41
   confrontation, 139
   immediacy, 139–40
   nondirectiveness, 140–41
   self-disclosure, 140–41
   summarizing, 141
religion and spirituality, 62–63
  of counselors, 62
  flexibility of beliefs, 62–63

not separating science from, 62
  by percentage in US, 62
REM (Reciprocal Engagement Model), 36–37, 126
Resta, Robert, 28, 29
RIAS (Roter Interaction Analysis System), 173
Richter, Melissa, 13, 24
Ritalin (methylphenidate), 55–56
Roberts, J. A. Fraser, 9, 11
Rogers, Carl, 15, 146, 147, 148
Roter, D., 173
Roter Interaction Analysis System (RIAS), 173
rubella, 9–10, 25
Rubin, Sylvia, 18

Sahhar, M., 79
Sarah Lawrence College, 13, 15–17, 24, 147
Schild, Sylvia, 11–12
schizophrenia, 55–56
self-awareness and self-knowledge, 2, 3, 43–44, 80–83
  audio-recording of sessions, 43–44, 82, 83
  countertransference, 81–82
  definition of, 80–81
  feminist therapy, 97–98
self-regulation theory, 180
SES (socioeconomic status), 47–48
Shkedi-Rafid, S., 93
sickle cell disease, 26, 98
Silver, J., 79
Singer, Niecee, 18
Smith, David, 8
Snyder, Laurence, 9, 10–11
Social Biology, 10
social cognitive theory, 182
social work, 11–12
Social Work and Genetics (Schild and Black), 11–12
socioeconomic status (SES), 47–48
solution-focused therapy. *See* problem-solving therapy
Spiridigliozzi, G. A., 93

spirituality. *See* religion and spirituality
Stanford Encyclopedia of Philosophy, 92
Stern, Alexandra Minna, 8, 12–13, 24
strength-based counseling, 164
  application to genetic counseling, 164
  theoretical concepts, 164
support and advocacy groups, 33–34
Suslak, Lorraine, 18
Syndromes of the Head and Neck (Gorlin and Pindborg), 8

Tannenbaum, Hody, 18
Targum, Steven, 12
Taylor, Shelley, 33–35
teach-back methods, 77–78
tele-genetic counseling and online genetic counseling, 174–75, 178–79, 194–95
Tenbrunsel, A. E., 117–18
teratogenic agents and counseling, 9–10, 100–1
thalidomide embryopathy, 9–10
Tips, Robert, 11–12
transactional theory of stress and coping, 180–81
transference and countertransference, 43, 46–47, 54, 81–82
  age difference between counselor and patient/client, 58
  conflicts of interest, 117
  counselors' personal and familial experiences, 58–59
Treasury of Human Inheritance, The (Pearson), 8–9
trisomy 18, 166

ultra-Orthodox Jewish patients and clients, 50, 63
ultrasonography, 13–14
University of California-Berkeley, 11–12, 15–16
University of California-Stanislaw, 83
University of Michigan, 9
University of Minnesota, 9
University of Pennsylvania, 113
University of Wisconsin, 90

utilitarian theories, 94–95
    counselor's application of, 94, 95
    premise of, 94
    theoretical scenario and, 94–95

virtue ethics, 95–96
    counselor's application of, 95–96
    premise of, 95
    theoretical scenario and, 95

Volkswagen Group, 114

Wallgren-Pettersson, C., 89
Warkany, Josef, 8
Weil, Jon, 12, 140–41
Wells Fargo Bank, 114
Wilson-Jungner criteria, 91

Yalom, Irvin, 146, 158–59

www.ingramcontent.com/pod-product-compliance
Ingram Content Group UK Ltd.
Pitfield, Milton Keynes, MK11 3LW, UK
UKHW022231230426
12048UKWH00016BA/1184